Viagra, Sex, and Romance

Copyright 1999, Boca Publications Group, Inc.

ISBN: 0-965-95831-0

Printed in Canada

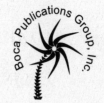

First published by Boca Publications Group
January, 1999

ALSO BY BOCA PUBLICATIONS GROUP:

CELINE DION: Behind The Fairytale

Viagra, Sex, and Romance

by

Elizabeth Myles

and

Bert MacFarlane

Acknowledgements

EDITOR, Esmond Choueke

COVER & PAGE DESIGN, Vadim Baboutin

LINE EDITOR, Catherine Arno

COVER MODEL, Debra Baker

PHOTO CONCEPT, Sorraya Wieneke

Cover photo copyright 1999 by Esmond Choueke

An original publication of:

BOCA PUBLICATIONS GROUP, INC.
7000 West Palmetto Park Rd., suite 400
Boca Raton, FL, USA, 33433

Please e-mail us at: BocaGroup@aol.com

ABOUT THE AUTHORS

ELIZABETH MYLES is a writer and researcher who specializes in topics involving relationships and emerging issues relevant to couples of all ages.

Her work has appeared in national and international publications. This is her first major book.

Having done a great deal of research into modern concepts of psychology, medicine, and the family, Ms. Myles believes that a frank and open discussion of the new eroticism can only benefit everyone in our society.

BERT MACFARLANE is a journalist who specializes in interviewing top medical experts around the world for articles in magazines and newspapers in the US, Canada, and Europe.

His articles often involve seeking out ordinary people with extraordinary stories to tell - many of which are included here.

INTRODUCTION

I've been deeply intrigued by the ways women and men are incorporating Viagra into the larger issues of love, relationships, and mutual sexual gratification. While the first wave of users were men, women have obviously discovered that it can work as an aphrodisiac for them as well.

Many of the stories from these couples are profound, touching, romantic, and beautiful, as well as being highly erotic.

These are the stories which we bring you in *Viagra, Sex, and Romance*

We sought out the best of these stories by interviewing users on phone chat lines, and by opening up a special e-mail address (**Aphrostory@aol.com**) where users were invited to send us their most memorable sexual experiences.

The erotic, emotional, and intellectual themes described by those interviewed have been maintained for our readers, while names and details were changed for confidentiality.

Some readers may object to the liberal use of "four-letter" words. However we feel they are essential to conveying these themes since they are the words used by those interviewed.

Our goal is to help our readers feel and understand how sexual and romantic experiences are evolving with libido-enhancing drugs including Viagra - which is only the first of many such products destined to appear in pharmacies in coming months.

Elizabeth Myles
January, 1999

Dear Readers...

If you would like to contribute an interesting story involving your intimate experiences with Viagra or any other sex-enhancement drug, we would appreciate hearing from you for the sequel to Viagra, Sex, & Romance.

Please e-mail the authors at: <u>*Aphrostory@aol.com*</u>

We'll send you a free copy of our next book if we use your contribution.

All names and places supplied will remain strictly confidential.

Best wishes,

Elizabeth Myles and Bert MacFarlane

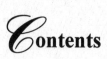ontents

DEDICATED TO all those who graciously shared their most intimate experiences with us and our readers.

Alyse's Adventure

SANDRA, MY FRIEND in the apartment below us, is the one who turned me on to Viagra. She read in *Cosmo* that they were doing clinical trials on women – and the women were reporting that it worked great on them. So, Sandra tried one of her husband's pills. She said it was like magic! She got so turned when her husband penetrated her that she felt she was being screwed by King Kong. She gave me a few of the pills to take home, and I agreed to swallow one on the night of my thirty-fifth birthday to see if anything special would happen for me too. Sandra says her husband needs the pill, but I know that my husband, Michael, doesn't. His hard-ons are really good and they last pretty long, and he always has a good orgasm inside me. I can tell because he makes these happy-sounding grunting and groaning noises whenever he's coming. He enjoys plain sex with my legs spread out for him so he can easily push his cock inside me. I do like that, but I'd be happy if it could be more orgasmic for me.

I knew Michael would want to have sex on my birthday since it was a special night, and I was a bit excited and nervous about what would happen to me on Viagra. I've hardly ever taken any kind of drug. Even when my friends in college were doing pot and other stuff, it never interested me. So I admit I was a bit scared. I didn't even tell Michael I had taken it. One reason was that I was afraid it might not do anything for me, and then I'd be embarrassed. Or, he might think I was starting to lose interest in him, or he might start to act self-conscious about his manhood. I guess I was just thinking *this is about me, not him, so let's give it a try.* And boy, was I happy I did.

We had planned to go into the city and take a sunset cruise around Manhattan for our celebration, and it turned out to be a really beautiful summer night. I put on my short black cocktail dress and I looked really cute, if I do say so. With my perky breasts, summer tan and bobbed dirty-blonde hair, I looked as sexy as I ever did when Michael and I started dating. When he saw me all done up, he teased me, saying, "You are my own, private, Ally McBeal - in fact, you're even cuter than she is." I don't think I look *that* much like her, but I liked the compliment. Michael looked pretty suave himself, with his curly dark hair, pale yellow shirt, and dark blue tie.

Sandra told me it would take about an hour for the Viagra to take effect, so I secretly took a half of my little blue pill when we ordered our first cocktail on the boat. Michael and I had a couple of margaritas as the boat began churning its way up the Hudson. It was certainly romantic to see all the lights of New York and New Jersey from the water, and Michael and I became really smoochie together. I mean, we've been married for seven years, and we have two kids, and we're not as sexy with each other as we used to be – so it was nice to be feeling basically quite horny about each other. But I was surprised when my vagina started feeling really different and very aroused - and I realized it must be the Viagra.

My pussy had never felt quite this way before. It had a powerful pulsating feeling inside it that seemed to pulse in time with my heartbeat. Soon, it also began feeling warmer both inside my vagina and on the outside on my clit and vulva. I felt so turned on I actually wanted to masturbate right then, and it took a lot of restraint to stop myself from sneaking off and reaching my own hand under my short black dress into my panties. I'm sure I could have made myself come within 30 seconds. It was really an exquisite feeling, and I wanted to make the most of it!

Michael and I wandered around on the upper deck as the sun set like a huge red ball. It began getting dark, and everybody else on board crowded around to watch the sun go down. I took Michael by the hand to the opposite side, and we stopped under the awning. I leaned against the railing with Michael facing me, and I couldn't stand it anymore. Nobody was able to see me because he was blocking any view of me, and, in any case they were staring at the sunset. I took his hand and made him reach under my dress stick his whole hand into my underpants right against my pussy. I told him, "Touch me, Michael, I want you to touch me now."

Michael was pretty surprised, and his eyes got really big like he couldn't believe what was happening. He said, "Ally, this is so neat, I guess I'm really turning you on tonight... I guess it's the flowers and love and all that... that's so great." I pretended to agree with him just to make sure he didn't stop what he was doing. He caught on fast, and continued rubbing his palm against my hot, wet pussy as I squirmed under his touch. I could see the backs of the other passengers as they leaned against the opposite railing, and I was thinking, *if only they knew how much fun I was having, they'd all be jealous!*

Michael wanted to kiss me and do some frenching inside my mouth, but I wasn't interested in that. All my attention was centered on my pussy, and the pounding sensation which was beginning to spread from the outside of my cunt back in through my vagina and into my whole body.

My heart was beating hard and fast, and I was breathing in fast gasps, and I was feeling so wonderful. He slipped a finger deep into me, and that made me see stars. I became totally lost in what I knew was going to be an amazing climax. After only about one single minute of Michael rubbing my clit with his hand and wriggling his finger inside me, I had a wet, gushing orgasm right into Michael's palm. I was careful not to make any sound or to change my expression in case anyone was watching us. Michael too pretended everything was normal, but I could tell he was really turned on by the whole experience. I brushed my hand against his groin, and I could feel his cock had grown very hard. I think the spontaneity of our encounter brought us both back to the time we first met and we couldn't keep our hands off each other. So far, my Viagra experience was great. And it would soon get even better!

I patted my dress down, and we turned around nonchalantly, acting as if nothing unusual had happened. He, of course, was still really horny – I could tell by the way he stayed close to me and rubbed my back as if he was hoping I'd start rubbing his cock. He was right that I wanted to, because I needed more pussy action to keep me happy that night. He even made extra compliments, like, "Ally, you're so sexy tonight... you feel so nice to me... I can't wait until I get to make love with you, darling." He didn't have to be so nice, I wanted him anyway.

We had another drink and some little appetizers they were handing out, and listened to the dj's music. By then it had grown completely dark, and I began touching Michael's cock from time to time when we were facing away from everybody else. I think his hard-on was getting bigger by the minute. I knew I was still having Viagra effects in my pussy, because it was more than ready to receive some extra attention!

Michael seemed to be growing desperate for some cock attention by then, and he told me, "Now, Ally, I need you now." He began leading me around to the other decks away from the other passengers and the waiters and waitresses, looking for a place where we'd be alone. The fact that I was turned on obviously turned him on! He tried opening a few doors marked DO NOT ENTER, and finally he found a small, dark equipment room – and shoved me quickly into it. It was as black as tar inside there, and we couldn't even see an inch in front of our faces. As soon as he closed the door, I unzipped Michael's trousers and stuck my hands down to caress his hot cock. His hands began groping under my dress, tugging at my panties and playing with my vagina. He kneeled down at my feet so he could pull my panties off, and while he was down there he put his face into my pussy and began licking it. I held him down with my hands and rubbed my clit and vulva up and down on his mouth and tongue until I came again. It was *so good* that I almost lost my breath.

I felt so naked and promiscuous – and excited. I said, "Yes, Michael, yes, I want your big cock inside me now, Michael, I want it in me now." And I really meant it.

We obviously couldn't take our clothes off in such a tiny area. He pulled his pants down to his thighs, then nudged my shoulders down in front of him so I'd blow him a little. I sucked on his hard-on, sliding my lips and tongue up and down his shaft. The Viagra had a special effect on my mouth as well as my vagina, because the feel of his cock on the inside of my cheeks and against my tongue was so vibrant. I stood back up, and he took my hips and turned me around backwards. I put my arms against the wall to steady myself, and I bent over a little so that my pussy would be at the same level as his cock. He rubbed my super-sensitive, totally wet vagina with his hand, and I became totally, steamy hot. He aimed his penis into me, and entered me easily and deeply from behind.

I felt him pumping his cock deep inside me, and the best part was the way the tip of it rubbed all the way up against my cervix. That made our secret fuck totally excellent. I love it when anything touches my cervix because it has always been one of my most sensitive erogenous areas, and that night it was twice as sensitive as ever. Michael's cock was poking at it over and over, giving me pulses of pure pleasure.

He began grasping at the cheeks of my ass and squeezing them tightly with his fingers, digging his nails into me, as if he wanted to make sure his penis was penetrating me to the maximum depth possible. Even the pain of his nails digging into my ass helped turn me on. In fact, I had never seen Michael so wild, and that was very flattering and sexy itself.

My cervix and the rest of my vagina began going ballistic. In a powerful series of bursts, my third orgasm exploded in me, even more wonderfully than the others. I was doubled up still with his cock in me from behind, and the walls of my vagina began vibrating around his cock like crazy. A raging, tingling feeling spread right through me from my clit all the way up to my ears, and I was suddenly coming in orgasmic waves. It was the most intense sensation I had ever experienced. I began unconsciously shaking my ass to get Michael's cock to rub every part of my pussy, and that made Michael come instantly, right after I did. His sperm shot deep inside me against my cervix, warm and wet. After climaxing like that, we were both gasping for air, trying to regain our composure following that overwhelming experience. When he finally pulled his cock out from behind me, I turned around and we clung to each other as if we had just run a marathon.

We both started laughing from the intensity of it all. Luckily, I had some tissues in my purse to soak up all the come, and we tried to make our clothes look normal so we could rejoin the tourists on the main part of the boat. He sneaked out first from the equipment room, and then so did I. Funny enough, he had put my panties in his pocket and forgot to return them. I certainly couldn't put them back on with everyone watching, so I spent the rest of the night with my vagina totally exposed beneath that little black dress. I think it was a good idea to let everything cool off down there after what I had been through!

I don't think anyone else on board noticed that we had been gone, but Michael and I had big secret smiles every time we glanced at each other.

* * * * *

Mavis

in

Cuba

ONE REASON I WENT TO CUBA for my vacation was because of the sexy Latino blokes they have there. I've admired their super-slim bodies and their café-au-lait skin in brochures and travel videos, and I love them all. They're so beautiful. I came to the conclusion that, as a 45-year-old stockbroker, I had better use my time and money to enjoy the pleasures I want before I became too old to appreciate them. My main craving in life is for totally dedicated sexual attention, and I felt that Cuba would be *the* place to get it. I also knew my money would go a long way there.

My ex took the kids for his week, and I left London on an organized tour to one of those Club Med type resorts with on-site activities and group dining and so on. But the activities

I had in mind weren't listed in our brochures. It turned out to be lucky for me that I found a reputable-looking pharmacy near the resort which was selling bottles of Viagra without prescription - because that little blue pill helped make my sexual adventure so volcanic.

I had heard a lot about Viagra, so I knew I wanted to try it to see if my sexual escapade would become super exciting. I was prepared to be fucked really well, and to come really well. In Britain, a lot of men don't give me a second look because I'm a little chubby, but Latino fellows seem to like that. At least I do have nice, large breasts which are a big plus anywhere.

Within a couple of days of hanging around on the beach I spotted the bloke I wanted most. He was working at the hotel as an activities organizer, and he also taught Latin dancing. I signed up for his dance classes immediately. His name was Carlos, and he was like a dream come true, like an Adonis. He was slim, but not skinny, with nicely defined muscles. He had a lovely face with full lips, dark eyes, and a smallish nose, all topped with a full head of thick, dark, wavy hair. He was a couple of inches shorter than I am, but I thought that made him cuter. And he was certainly younger than me, by about 20 years! I also admired him because he was very well educated, with a degree in chemistry. But, there was so little work in his field that he had to work in the tourist industry.

As he taught us the moves to the marengue, conga and salsa, I couldn't stop drooling over him. The music was playing and he was taking turns with all the women to show them the right steps. All I could focus on were his great hips and his fantastic round ass which swayed beautifully to the Latin rhythms. When it was my turn to dance with him, I held him tightly so I could feel the sensuous movements of his body, and so I could press my breasts against him to get him to notice me. In his cute Spanish accent he was saying, "Feel the music, Mavis, feel it in your hips." I could hardly bear to let him leave after our dance! My heart was beating fast, telling me to hang on to him all night. But, more planning was needed to figure out how to end up alone with him.

My chance came the next night as all the male and female activity coordinators put on a fashion show for the guests. Carlos and the other models took turns walking down the runway showing off the vacation clothing that was on sale in the hotel boutique. He was modeling a tennis outfit with bright white shorts and shirt, both with turquoise trim and monograms of the hotel. As he walked I was so taken by the whole image of him that my head began to spin. I was able to see his penis bulging behind the zipper, and I felt my heart and my vagina bursting with desire to have him as soon as humanly possible.

During the break in the show, I moved over beside him to start chatting a bit. He was very friendly to me and seemed to like me, but frankly, I think he knew I'd be able to provide him with some extra cash if he'd hang out with me. I didn't really care what his motives were as long as he was with me. After all, he was beautiful, and it was my holiday. Also, it was obvious that the people in Cuba are quite poor, so if I could make him or his family happier by spreading some money around, what's wrong with that? I'm sure he wouldn't have hung out with me if he didn't care for me at all. And I was also sure he appreciated my bosom from the glances he made towards my chest.

It was forbidden for him to be too close to guests in the hotel, and he was quite scared of losing his job. So, I suggested to him, "Carlos, why don't you show me some of the wild discos I've heard about in Havana? I'll be happy to take you as my guest." So, after the fashion show we actually left together for downtown Havana. We had a few drinks while a great Latino band played, and I took one of the little blue pills, hoping it would be a lucky night for me.

Soon, we were dancing the salsa so close I could feel his penis and thigh muscles brushing against my upper leg. "Well, Mavis," Carlos said, "I see you've learned something from our dance lessons."

The Viagra must have been working full-speed ahead, because my clit and my nipples became so sensitive I thought I'd have an orgasm right there on the dance floor. I simple had never felt so horny and wild and crazy before. *This is sexual desire as it should be*, I thought. I knew I had to have his penis in my vagina and in my mouth that very night. I asked him rather audaciously, "Would you like to be alone with me for awhile?" and he accepted with a nod. I simply rented another hotel room downtown so we could go there to screw.

That first sexual episode with Carlos was a time I'll never forget. As soon as we were alone, we both took off all our clothes. Seeing him totally naked with his beautiful hips and his cock - which was hard and long and thick - at my disposal was pure bliss. He obviously didn't mind my being a little overweight. And, even though I've always been embarrassed about my nipples because they're rather large and flat, he didn't mind that either. In fact, he said he liked my breasts because they were so big and soft, and he licked and squeezed them continually, which was fine with me. He didn't go in much for cunnilingus, but I didn't care because I'm a big fan of true fucking with a nice firm cock – which was something my ex-husband was hardly ever able to deliver.

Carlos and I had been sweating quite a lot from the heat and the dancing, and when we embraced we were slipping and sliding all over each from our total body moistness. He told me he didn't have any diseases, so I let him make love to me without a condom. My legs and my pussy were trembling with desire and I couldn't wait for him to shove his nice hard erection into me. I lay down on my back, grabbed his firm, round ass with both hands and brought his hips and cock down against my eagerly-awaiting, super-wet crotch.

His hard-on was firm as a plantain as he slid into my pussy. He began gyrating in me, and it made me feel totally wild. The dinky radio on the night-table was playing non-stop salsa, and Carlos was swaying his hips and humping me smoothly and rhythmically if he was dancing to the beat with his cock. His penis was rubbing my labia, my clit, and my G-spot to that salsa beat, and, with the Viagra pulsing through my vagina, I realized my pussy had become transformed into an automatic orgasm-generator. I reached my first climax within minutes, and then I came over and over again. I had never experienced multiple orgasms like that before, and it was a deeply-satisfying spiritual and physical ecstasy.

Carlos never stopped screwing me even after he came the first time, and he stayed hard and kept on humping me until he had his second orgasm. Meanwhile, I was experiencing my own pulsing, engulfing orgasms, and it felt wonderful to have him continue screwing me even during and after my climaxes.

Having Carlos's cock inside me and knowing he was using my vagina to come twice in a row made me feel more sexually satisfied than I ever had in my entire life. To me, it was far better than any dumb romantic gestures that any man had ever made towards me, like sending flowers or paying for dinner. This is what showed he really cared and appreciated me as a woman. I liked the fact that me and my vagina turned Carlos on so much. I liked feeling my vagina overflowing with his hot, sticky come. I wanted my vagina to be used like that. It made me feel like a total woman.

When we finally took a break, I was as limp and wet as a rag doll that had been tossed around in a tornado! My orgasms had taken so much energy out of me that I could barely move. I felt like I had reached a sexual Nirvana through my Viagra orgasms. It was a height of pleasure I had never known before.

Carlos and I both were totally smeared with my juices and his, and all of our pores emanated the heady smell of sex which enveloped us like a cloud.

Eventually we struggled into the shower, and we lazily rubbed handfuls of soapsuds over every inch of each other. The lights were on bright since there were no shades on the bulbs, and he enjoyed seeing and playing with my large white breasts. He also seemed to like the extra roundness of my tummy and rear end. I felt wild when he reached down to soap up my pussy and ass. I could barely get enough of him. I filled my hands with soapsuds and squeezed my fingers right in between the cheeks of his ass, his anus, then all over his testicles, and around his now-resting penis. It wasn't long before he got hard again, and I was back in bed in the missionary position with his lovely cock swaying inside me again.

At the end of the evening, I put $200 US into his pocket, and we made plans to meet again during the week.

The only trouble was, my pussy had seen more action that one night than I had experienced during months of being married, and it really wore me out. So, I only felt comfortable booking a night with Carlos one more time when my vagina had recovered.

Carlos actually flirted with me a bit every day when we encountered each other at the club, and that was very flattering. I actually toyed with the idea of bringing him back home with me - he would have made a better husband than my ex, I bet. I thought I could try to find him a job using my connections... but those daydreams were just my silly girlish nature coming out.

Before my second date with Carlos, I took another one of my pills, and I enjoyed our sexual activity as much as the first time. It turned out to be the best holiday I've ever had.

Since that trip, I've thought about Carlos a lot, and he attempts to write to me occasionally in his halting English. I've told several of my girlfriends about it all. Surprisingly, none of them has taken me up on the idea of doing a trip together, but I'm sure I'll be heading down there again soon.

* * * * *

Viagra, Sex, & Romance

Bradley

Breaks Free

I'M 16 AND MY PENIS DOESN'T work very well for sex because of a bike accident I had two years ago. I was zooming down a hill, hit a rock, and my quick-release front wheel popped right off. I tried to hang onto the bike as the wheel went flying, and I ended up smashing my testicles and penis really hard down onto the metal frame as everything busted up. The pain was terrible. But worse than that, I also squished and damaged that spongy material inside a penis which fills up with blood and lets you have erections. That's how my urologist explained it to me. He said my cock might start to produce better erections as I got older, but so far it hasn't.

I like girls just like other guys do, and I've had a girlfriend now for more than a year. She's also 16. But sex has been a problem until I got some Viagra pills. I want to tell you about it because of other guys who may be having the same problem as me.

When my girlfriend Vanessa and I used to make out, I would get mini-erections which were always kind of soft and could go away at any time. I used to hate to get naked because my erection wasn't strong and hard like it's supposed to be.

I do love seeing her get naked, even if my cock doesn't respond. She's a redhead with long straight hair and amazing curly red cunt hair between her white legs. She also has lots of freckles all over her white skin, so all of that together makes her totally stunning. She smells really nice too, like a mix between deodorant and perfume. She never has any strong smell on her pussy. She lets me touch her everywhere, and I get to finger her and play with her until she comes. I can make her come pretty easily because of her directions, like, "Slower, Bradley, deeper, Bradley," and so on.

I've done oral sex on her a few times and it's neat for me to put my face into her cunt and lick it, with her red curlies rubbing against my lips. She likes that too, of course.

Meanwhile, to try to do something for me, Vanessa would stick her hands in my jeans and to give me a hand-job. Sometimes it would work and sometimes it wouldn't. She's a good sport about it and doesn't make fun of me. But I was sure she'd want to try having intercourse sooner or later because everyone in school talks about it all the time. In fact, loads of kids are already doing it. I definitely wanted to be able to have intercourse, and I wanted Vanessa and I to lose our virginity together.

Everyone began hearing about the Viagra stuff, and I asked my doctor about it. He was pretty cool, and got me a prescription of it to try out and even wished me luck. And it made my whole life better. Like he told me, I take a pill a little while before we plan to try intercourse, and pretty soon, my hard-ons begin to appear. And they really are hard, all the way along my cock from the bottom to the top. And my cock sometimes stays hard for awhile even after I come, so I can come again. It's like totally great.

The first time Vanessa and I had successful sex was one day after school at her house, right on her parent's bed. We planned everything just right. I took the pill as we were walking home from school. I could feel something good happening almost right away. My penis got hard right inside my pants, and it stayed hard as we walked and talked. "It's working, Vanessa, it's working!" I whispered in her ear. She had a big smile. We knew her parents wouldn't be home for at least a few hours, so we headed straight for their bed, which is the biggest bed in the house.

We both took off our clothes right away, and there we were, both totally naked – and me with my erection. I was pretty proud of it and I thought, *I'm normal, this is excellent, I'm just like all the guys. Now it's time to use it!*

We didn't use a condom because we wanted to have the full experience of sex for our first time, and we knew neither of us had an STD or AIDS because we've never had sex before anyway. We figured Vanessa could take the morning-after pill the next day in case she got pregnant.

I could hardly wait to see how my cock would feel inside her vagina. She lay back on the pillows with her knees up, and I fingered her a little to get her lubricated for me. Meanwhile, she was gripping my hard-on, saying, "Bradley - it's awesome!"

I moved my hips up towards her face, and aimed my penis in her mouth and man – that was great. I never used to want her to do oral sex on me because she tried it once or twice and my cock just didn't get hard, and I was really embarrassed. But this time I had so much sexy feeling in my cock that I could have shot off right in her throat, like you're supposed to with oral sex. The Viagra not only made me hard, it also made my cock feel really sensitive and horny. I took my cock away from her lips, saying, "Vanessa, I think this is the time, and I want to tell you I love you - and that I'm going to squeeze my boner right into your pussy!" Vanessa helped a little by lifting up her knees and spreading her legs a little. She was really wet by then so I was able to start sliding my cock right in. And we both started laughing with relief that everything was working.

Vanessa was saying, "Oh yes, oh yes, Brad, I really want you to, I really love you, I really want you in me."

I started going in pretty slowly. I was glad we kept the lights on because I loved watching my boner entering her cunt through her red curlies. Her vagina felt pretty hot on the end of my penis, which was sliding in nicely. I didn't want to push it in too fast because I had that feeling that I was going to come any second, and I wanted to make it last as long as I could.

I got in halfway, and then we both found out she had a hymen, or part of one. I pushed against it with the end of my cock, and I could feel it like a tight rubber band preventing my penis from entering her. I pushed a few times, and she started to cry. I knew I was hurting her, but she said, "It's okay, Brad, keep going, it's okay." I really did want to get in all the way, and I realized I need a really hard push. Actually, my erection felt so stiff and strong, I knew I could do it.

I was still lying on top of her, and I lifted up body onto my toes and elbows as if I was doing a push-up. Then I lowered my hips down with all my weight on my cock. *That* forced my erection hard into her vagina all the way to the point where I came up against her hymen. There was a squidgy sound and a feeling like a rubber band stretching around my hard-on and then breaking, and I popped right through her hymen. I was suddenly all the way deep into Vanessa's vagina. She yelped in pain, but started laughing with me through her tears.

I was so excited I yelled out, "I'm in! I did it, we're totally screwing!"

And said with a smile, "We're not virgins anymore! I love you so much, Brad!" And I told her I loved her too.

By then, my cock had been inside her for several minutes, and I was afraid to move even the tiniest bit because I knew the slightest movement would make me come. I felt so hot and sexy for the first time in my life. I couldn't really keep myself back from pumping my cock. I loved the great new feeling I was having. I moved a little, and I could feel the walls of her vagina clinging tight around my hard-on. A few seconds more and I reached an amazing climax where my cock felt like it was exploding. I had an orgasm deep inside her, and it felt so fantastic, like I was shooting off into a deep dark, cave hidden within Vanessa's soul.

When I pulled out my cock, she rubbed her cunt a little to try to get rid of the soreness. Pretty soon she stopped crying and all, and I even got another hard-on. So back I went into her, and it was better than the first time because she wasn't crying any more.

She even got on top of me for a while, and it looked to me like she was riding a teeter-totter on my hips. It was a view of her I never had before, and it was completely cool. I came again, and I was really happy about it because it was proof that my cock was working the way it's supposed to. For the first time since my bike accident, I didn't feel like a freak. I realized that if my cock didn't start to produce hard-ons on its own, that I could still always use Viagra to get it going when I wanted.

Vanessa's red curlies were now all really, really gooey from all the come I had shot off into her, so we went together to have a shower. I loved helping her suds up her cunt with body shampoo, and we hugged and all under the hot rushing water. It definitely was one of the best days of my whole life. We lay down for a while to watch TV, and I played with her clit as I usually do until she came. I wanted to make sure she was really happy too.

I don't know what other kinds of injuries you can fix up with Viagra, but to me it's like a miracle.

* * * * *

Maxine's

Second

Honeymoon

MY HUSBAND KENNETH AND I were dying to take a real vacation together. It seemed as if our entire lives for the first 12 years of marriage were dedicated to raising our two kids and working all day to pay their bills. It was time to have some fun and do something for *us*. As soon as our second child became more independent, we decided to have a second honeymoon at the same place we had our first one more than a decade ago – Niagara Falls. We just wanted to have a great time and feel young and happy again.

Part of our plan was to make sure that this honeymoon would be as sexy and hot as our first one, so I agreed to go along with Kenny's plan for us to both take Viagra. I don't know if it's true or not, but Kenny told me the drug was

34

Viagra, Sex, & Romance

named Viagra because it rhymes with Niagara, so that was an extra reason for both of us to take it there. I actually thought Viagra got its name because it sounds like vagina, and I think I'm right. In any case, I was reading about how it can make a woman become more orgasmic by increasing the sensitivity of her clitoris and vagina, and that sounded good to me. This was going to be the perfect opportunity for me to try it out. Kenny and I already knew it worked on him.

For the past couple of years, Kenny hasn't been doing very well in the sex department. He always complained that he had too much work to do, that he was tired, that sex made him more tired, and that I nagged him too much. It was, "Maxine, I love you more than ever, but I'm a little bit under the weather now because of our Asian contract." Or, "Maxine, let's concentrate on getting a good night's sleep so we can do it better tomorrow." That kind of crap.

All of these were excuses for why we hardly ever had sex anymore. At most it would be once or twice a month. And, he always rushed though the foreplay, I think, because he'd be nervous his penis wouldn't stay hard long enough. Once in a while his penis wouldn't work at all, and he might give me oral sex as a substitute. I enjoy his tongue-induced orgasm, and it's a rush to have his lips, mouth, and moustache caressing my vulva. But I started to feel bad for him if he didn't get an erection, and that made me avoid initiating sex.

Kenny went to a psychologist who explored his past and asked him all sorts of questions about his mother and his anxieties, but none of that made his penis hard. It took Viagra to do that. A urologist gave him a prescription for the 100 mg tablets, and it worked wonders for him immediately. Every time he took one, he got nice and hard. But, even though he could screw me nicely, there was just no romance behind it.

I figured that taking Viagra with him would get me on the same wavelength as him and that it would help us understand each other better.

So, that weekend, we shipped the kids off to his brothers' and drove up to the falls from Pennsylvania. Once we arrived, we arranged our schedule to repeat some of the same things we did 12 years earlier. I was hoping – and I think Kenny was too - that being in the same places would bring back the same magic we had felt back then. And, that would get us screwing like crazy. We even booked into one of those honeymoon hotels with our own jacuzzi and lots of mirrors everywhere.

The first night we just hit the sack because we were too tired from driving to even think about sex or touring. We slept in late the next morning, then started out on The Maid of the Mist boat tour that swings right beside the foot of the falls – exactly where we had been on our first honeymoon. Kenny was very attentive and put his arm around me, and we kissed from time to time with the spray of the falls sprinkling our faces. After that beautiful ride we walked through the tacky souvenir stores for an hour, and bought some stuff for the kids. When we sat down for a coffee break, Kenny took one of his 100-mg Viagra pills and broke another one in half for me to take.

"So, Kenny - you think you might get lucky today?" I teased him. I looked him in the eye as I swallowed my Viagra.

Kenny answered, "Maybe *you're* going to be the one who's lucky, Maxine." And he was more than right. We returned to our hotel, tossed some bubble bath into our jacuzzi, and the action started almost right away. We kept the lights on, and I began taking off my clothes. It was quite interesting, because I realized Kenny was staring at me in the multiple mirrors. I was being reflected everywhere - on the ceiling, the walls everywhere. I looked pretty good, actually. I took off my blouse, and I was happy I had put on a lacy pink bra that morning because it was very pretty against my skin. My breasts are small, at 32B, but they're also very firm and youthful looking. I'm almost as slim as I was when we married, so overall I'm a pretty nice package. I could see Kenny in the mirrors as he was watching me, and, from the moment he dropped his drawers, he had a nice, big hard-on.

He came into the jacuzzi right after me, and he floated me over to his lap. I straddled his legs and he began tonguing me in my mouth, and the licking and sucking on my breasts. Normally that really turns me on since my breasts are very sensitive. But the Viagra was making my whole body sexually receptive that afternoon. It felt as if my breasts were sending messages down to my clit to make me feel more orgasmic with every touch. That day was super-breast-day. Each time he licked or sucked my nipples, sparks of ecstasy rippled through me. As I floated on his lap with my vagina brushing up against his belly button we looked at each other with feelings of love.

The weird thing was, his erection was pressing against my rear end in between my legs, and the tip of his cock was kind of tickling my anus. I felt overwhelmingly sensitive in the middle of my ass and I wriggled up against his penis. I know the sensitivity was coming from the affects of the Viagra because I had never felt that way before, and it felt really good. I was very curious as to what was going to develop.

Kenny had never stimulated me much in that area ever before except for the fact that from time to time during intercourse he'd rub my anus a bit with his little finger. Now, as the tip of his penis rubbed against me there, it sent shivers of excitement through my whole body. Each time I felt his penis poking against me, I'd wiggle my buttocks to see if that would help him start to enter me. I think Kenny was as surprised as I was when that did start happening. I mean, we had talked about anal sex before, but we had never actually done it. I was becoming desperate to have him push his cock deep into my ass. I had a feeling it would hurt, but in an extremely pleasureful way. So, I kept lightly tapping my anus against the tip of his cock to see if it would start to come deeper inside me.

The water was already quite soapy and slippery from the bubble bath, and I could feel him trying hard to stick his cock in further. It was the most exotic feeling I had ever experienced. I knew we needed more lubrication if he was going to get in all the way as I wanted him to. So, I leaned over and grabbed one of the hotel's little bottles of hand cream and squeezed a gob of it onto my palm. I reached right under the water and rubbed it around Kenny's very manly cock with both hands as he lay back and purred at my attentions.

I straddled him again and put my breast back in his mouth. He held my hips in his hands to guide me, and this time his erection found its mark between my buttocks and began a slow, steady ascent into my anus. I was relaxed and hot, and I let him penetrate me as deeply as possible. It was like being a virgin again, as I had never felt these feelings before. In a way, I felt as if my hymen was being broken. Luckily, the cream I had smeared on his cock allowed him to slide in with almost no pain. His steady, piercing journey deep into my anus made me feel as if his cock was filling up my entire body, bringing me an excruciating type of pleasure.

Finally, his cock settled into me and he began slowly rotating his hips. I could tell he was super-excited. His pulse was beating so hard I could even feel it vibrating in his penis.

Along with sucking my nipples and fucking my ass, Kenny was also rubbing my bush with his hands and fingers. My vulva and clit were swollen with an aching desire, and I would have been happy to keep those super sexy feelings going all night. But my own level of Viagra-induced excitement mounted higher and higher, and I knew I'd never be able to stop the super-powerful orgasm that was building up within me from bursting forth. I was delirious with the thought that I'd be coming soon. Like a mini-explosion inside me, my orgasm began to overtake my consciousness, and my anus and vagina were shuddering with pulses of ecstasy which shook my whole body. I was *screaming* with pleasure and I didn't care! It was impossible for me to be ladylike when my vagina was going insane!

Kenny began going wild a moment after I began. He shot out his come deep into my ass, grabbing onto my cheeks with all his strength to keep himself deep within me. He had the most intense orgasm I had seem him have in years, and he was making a surprisingly sexy, growling, primeval sound as he climaxed.

My anus was still tight around the base of his cock, so it remained erect until he slowly pulled it out of me. *Then,* it was time for a rest. We both flopped back against the side of the jacuzzi and let the powerful streams of water massage our genitals as we lay there exhausted. It took a while for us to get our breath back, and finally we turned and looked at each other incredulously. We both smiled and then began laughing at the thought of the experience we just had. I wondered how we'd ever be able to top it.

Later on, we dried off, had a nap, and then went out to look for a restaurant. The falls were illuminated with different colored lights, and it was quite beautiful walking together in the starry night with that beautiful view spread out in front of us. "Maxine, I don't think it gets much better than this," Ken said, and it felt like we were back on our first honeymoon. We were starting to feel that we belonged to each other again.

We ate a lovely surf-and-turf dinner of grilled scampi with lemon and basil, and filet mignon with mushroom sauce, and polished off a nice bottle of Cavernay Sauvignon before sauntering back to our room. We were lying in bed reminiscing about our first honeymoon when Kenny turned over onto me, his cock once again hard as a rock, and he began penetrating me right in my pussy. I don't know if there were lingering effects from the Viagra making us horny, or if we were just so turned on by each other we didn't need any extra boost – but I was so ready for him, it was wonderful. He looked deeply into my eyes and fucked me nice and slowly, and we tongue-wrestled for the longest time. I rubbed my clit a little with my fingers because it felt so good, and I came within five minutes. He wanted to have his way with me, so he kept screwing me for the longest time after I came, and then he ejaculated into my pussy groaning into my ear as he always used to do. I loved hearing that.

The next day we toured the Houdini Museum on the way out to dinner. In one of the darkened areas where Houdini's magical illusions were on display, Kenny was standing behind me and he began massaging my breasts from behind. It was pretty obvious what he had on his mind. At the water fountain, he slipped me the remaining half of my Viagra pill, and I gulped it down while he took another whole one himself.

I wondered what we would be up to next. I found out a little later when he played a funny magic trick on me! He had told me not to wear any underwear under my low-cut wrap-around dress when we went out, and it made me feel sexy to oblige. As we walked to a nice Italian restaurant, I could feel the air circulating under my dress, blowing on my vagina, and I felt naked and excited. By the time we were seated, we were both having hot thoughts, and we began paying a lot of attention to each other. He'd brush aside the top of my dress to look at my breast when nobody was watching. As for me, I slipped off my high heels and began playing with his crotch with my bare toes under the table when the waitress wasn't around.

After our dinner arrived, I playfully lifted up my foot to play with his crotch one last time before eating, and I found my toes squeezing against his bare-naked erection! He had secretly unzipped his fly without my noticing, and there was his cock, standing up at attention underneath the tablecloth. That was such a cute trick I almost burst out laughing. It made me feel so special that he went to all that trouble. I just wanted to jump under the table, kneel down at his feet, and suck on his hard-on like Julie Christie did to Warren Beatty in the movie Shampoo. But, unfortunately, I had to hold myself back since we were in a very public place!

We had a lovely tiramisu for dessert, then went out for a stroll in the cool night air. We decided to take the pedestrian path across the Rainbow Bridge which joins to Canada, and it was a real experience being above the water like that. Nobody else was around because it was pretty late. I looked at Kenny and I said, "Kenny, let's always remember how much fun we can have just being alone with each other." As we walked on the metal structure, we could feel the bridge vibrating under our feet as cars crossed over it. The sensation made us laugh nervously. I actually was a bit scared. I never knew that a big bridge could bounce and sway like that just from cars driving by.

When we reached a third of the way across I had enough and wanted to turn back. Kenny said, "Maxine - I think there's a toll for using this bridge, and that means a big, big kiss." Of course I was happy to kiss him, and it was quite delicious. I was leaning backwards against the railing, and he was pressing close to me when I felt that old magic trick coming back – he had unzipped himself, and his erection was pressing against my crotch. Now I knew why he didn't want me to wear any underwear that night! We hadn't had sex standing up for years. My vagina was really geared up by the Viagra boost and by those romantic memories swirling through my mind. I really wanted Kenny to get his cock inside me, and fast! The way we were situated made it impossible for anyone to see what we were up to. So I lifted up my dress, grabbed his erect penis, and rubbed it against my clitoris and vulva to spread my pussy lubrication around.

A minute later, the tip of Kenny's cock was sliding into me between my tingling vulva. Since he's a bit taller than I am, the top of his cock was rubbing against my clitoris, and with all that stimulation I could feel the pressure of an orgasm growing stronger and stronger really quickly inside my vagina. For me, anyway, I was about to have the thrill of a great, quick, zipless fuck, and I shook my hips and pussy fast and hard against his cock to make myself come as soon as possible. Kenny was lifting my thighs in a tight grip to maintain our fucking position and he was using his fingers to tickle my most sensitive erogenous spot, the little area right between my vagina and anus.

I was so into my own excitement that for once I wasn't thinking about Kenny's orgasm at all. I wanted him to keep doing me as fast as possible just so I could be released with an orgasm. Before I knew it, the pleasure within my crotch spread through me and I felt a huge, quick series of shockwaves from my vagina growing into one of the most powerful, pounding orgasms I had ever experienced. Kenny could hardly last much longer. I felt his grip tighten on my thighs as he loudly began groaning in time to the surges of his own sperm.

What a night that was, screwing on that swaying bridge with the falls rushing in the distance. It was better than my wildest dreams, and was a great honeymoon in *every* sense of the word.

I guess we'll slowly end up returning to our old, normal routine again once we get back home. But it's good to know we can get away together and have a romantic and sexual adventure anytime we want and renew our spiritual connection.

* * * * *

Daltry

the

Trucker

I'M A TRUCKER NAMED DALTRY, and I haul furniture around the country. I help load the vans in one city, and then help unload them in another. Doing this kind of work plays hell with your mind and body. Half the time you're driving through the middle of the night, half the time you're trying to doze in the tiny bed at the back of the cab. You never eat right, and you're always in a rush as you press the pedal to the metal down endless highways. I was so whacked out most of the time that I could barely keep my eyes open when my wife and I were together or when I was supposed to take care of our little girls. The only thing I ever wanted to do when I was home was to lie around and sleep. As far as sex went, I was almost totally *kaput*. I didn't have the energy for it anymore, even though I loved my wife. That was why she and I broke up. She said simply, "Daltry, this isn't even a marriage anymore." And it looked like she was right.

The thing is, I didn't know what other kind of work I ever could do to keep a roof over our heads. I had no choice but to keep on working for this moving company even though my wife, Geraldine, was getting fed up. She warned me many times, but I didn't think she was so pissed off that she'd actually leave me. She said, finally, that if she had to do everything alone all of the time, she might as well be alone. It really tore me apart when we separated, and I begged her not to. She said, "You know, Daltry, it's not how much you love me and need me that counts, it's the way we live our lives."

Being alone for many weeks made me think a lot. I became more and more determined to try to win Geraldine back - and Viagra helped me do it.

I first had a few long talks with Geraldine's mom, and I asked her for her advice and help in trying to figure out what I could do. I was grateful that she took me seriously and helped me work out various plans that I hadn't considered. She and I came up with the idea that I'd take one entire week off each month even though it meant I'd make that much less pay. During that week, I could be a totally devoted family man, and I'd still be able to keep my job.

The next step was to convince Geraldine to take me back so we could try out my new work schedule together. I said, "Geraldine, please, we'll see really quickly if my new plan improves our family life and makes you more satisfied with having me. Those are the biggest goal of my life right now." With her mother backing me up, Geraldine did agree to have me move in on a trial basis, and I set about to make our first week together really romantic for both of us.

Viagra, Sex, & Romance

To tell the truth, I was worried about the fact that I wasn't much of a stud anymore since I was so wrecked from work. At the best of times, we were lucky if we'd make love once a month. Half the time Geraldine would try to suck my cock to make it go up so that we could have sex - but it would hardly go up at all. I certainly don't blame her for resenting me about that, even though we didn't discuss it much. The sexual aspect of our life would surely have to improve to make us feel more romantic towards each other - and if we were going to succeed as a married couple.

On a lark, I decided to take one-and-a-half Viagra pills (that's a total of 150 mg) each time because I'm so big, at 210 pounds and six feet tall - and it really did the trick for me. I don't mean to brag, but I've always had the largest cock in my gang. When erect, it's more than six inches long, and it gets really thick like a heavy gear shift lever. So, I figured I'd need an extra powerful dose to get my gun reloaded when the time was right. That first week when we started living together again, I took it every day. And, by the end of the week, I had Geraldine loving me so much that it almost hurt both of us.

I acted kind of shy the first night we got back together, offering to sleep on the couch. She said I might as well sleep in bed with her, because nothing was going to happen anyway. Was she ever surprised! She turned over to go to sleep, not expecting any sex since she hadn't even tried to touch my cock. But it had become magnificently erect, just like it used to when Geraldine and I were first married. My boner was hot for action, and I was hoping for a truly romantic union.

I didn't want to be too aggressive, so, without saying a word, I slowly leaned down under the covers and began doing oral sex on her, licking her vagina in swirls, the way she used to like. I could feel her hips begin grinding up into my face, and I knew she was getting really turned on. As for myself, my nice, hard erection was ready, willing, and able to go into action whenever Geraldine decided the time was right. She moaned and groaned with each lick of my tongue, and, finally, she slid her hand down towards my cock, probably figuring she'd have to do her regular suck-on-me routine. But she found that hard-as-steel stick-shift of mine, and she was happy. She said, "I guess this means you missed me, Daltry..." and I replied that I surely did.

Geraldine didn't even try to suck me. She just climbed on top of me and aimed my erection into her wet vagina. By then my hard-on had grown into its full potential and was as big, wide and hard as ever. She had a hard time squeezing her cunt down onto it. Her pussy felt tight and sexy as she wiggled it around to get it to accept my cock. Finally, she sank all the way down, and my cock felt like it was in the place where it belonged forever.

Geraldine began humping me like there was no tomorrow. I guess she was worried that my hard-on would squish up like it had been doing in the past year, so she wanted to take advantage of it as long as it stayed hard. Little did she know that I was going to have giant boners like that every night of our first week back together, thanks to my little blue pills!

I began fondling her breasts and her butt, and squeezing her nipples in my fingers the way she used to like it. She got super-excited, and she humped even faster as she was about to climax, and the tip of my cock started to feel like it was being whipped by lightening. She began shuddering and moaning as she had a big orgasm, then lay on my chest for only a minute before starting to hump me again. She kept right on going like the Eveready bunny. I guess she was hoping to keep using my

Viagra, Sex, & Romance

nice boner for as long as she could - especially because she had been deprived of good sex because of me for so long.

This time, Geraldine reached down to her clit and rubbed it for a minute to bring herself to her second orgasm. Those jittery motions of hers when she climaxed set me off too – and I began shooting my load into her a moment later. My hard-on was pointing straight up into her cunt, and my shot felt like a rocket roaring off a launch pad. Geraldine obviously noticed what a great orgasm I was having since my whole body began rocking, and because I was making loud grunting noises. She asked jokingly, "Does this mean you really did miss me?" I always did like her sense of humor.

As soon as I recovered from my orgasm, I told her simply that I always had loved her since the first day I met her, and that I still loved her just as much. She replied, "Daltry, please don't let your emotions get ahead of you because there's been a lot of water under the bridge. Let's just take everything one day at a time. I agreed, but I still took the Viagra every day, as I had planned. And we fucked like crazy that whole week.

I felt very confident about my hard-ons, and that's what gave me the guts to fuck her wherever and whenever I could. When the kids were at school in the afternoon, we boinked on the kitchen counter and on the velvet couches in the den. I also bent her backwards over the washing machine, and fucked her standing up.

On our last night together before I took off for my truck route again, I took my sixth Viagra dose of the week, and I was really glad I did. Much to my surprise, Geraldine sauntered into our bedroom dressed up in a super sexy green baby-doll outfit complete with matching see-through panties and top, and with ruffles and bows all over the place. She said,

"Daltry, I really appreciate the effort you've made this week to be together with all of us and to be a good guy. Now, I'm going to give *you* something to remember me by during your next shift."

I got so excited at the sight of my wife in that horny outfit that my cock jacked up to attention. I said, "Don't worry baby, there's no way I'm going to forget this sight..."

I wanted to fuck her so badly I barely hugged her or kissed her before I pulled off my pj's and began rubbing my hard-on against her pussy. Geraldine just said, "Do me, Daltry, do me like you did the first night you came back..." and I did. I had her lie down on her back with her knees up and her cunt peeking up at me through that sheer green pair of panties, glistening with anticipation as if it had a mind of its own. I licked her cunt through the material to excite her, and a few of her pubic hairs started poking through, tickling my tongue. I was laughing from that and I told her why, and she began laughing too. We were starting to be a romantic couple again, I hoped!

We got into a position to do 69 together, and, while I continued licking her through the panties, she began to suck as much of my cock as she could fit into her mouth. She rubbed the bottom part of my cock with her hand, and then licked my bag and my balls. She made me the horniest I had been for the whole week, and I could hardly stand it anymore. I needed to fuck her cunt! I got on top of her and got my big boner into her. I began screwing her wild and wet pussy firmly and slowly so that we could both feel as much sensation as possible for as long as possible. I didn't want it to end!

Geraldine really got into my rhythms too, and she began grunting in time to my fucking. It was a long, slow, deep fuck, and even after I came, my boner stayed big and I fucked her some more. I felt like I could have screwed her the whole night through, and I kept on going until she shook in my arms and climaxed in a stunning rush.

Geraldine said, "So, you're the sexy animal I married... and I'm happy that you're *my* sexy animal." She was right - I was totally hers in any form she wanted. I was so glad that my plan of action was succeeding with my romantic moves, my Viagra, and my changes at work. I was grateful for the chance to be able to stay married to Geraldine, and whatever it takes to stay married, that's what I'll do.

* * * * *

the *Widow*

Yolanda

I USED VIAGRA TO SEDUCE a younger man, and it was a fantastic experience.

My name is Yolanda, and I'm a 62-year-old widow. My husband died two years ago, and it was the worst thing I've ever been through. He had always been so loving and so caring towards me. I knew I'd never find that again in a man. I just cried my eyes out for weeks on end. I even had hallucinations that he was visiting me at night, at the foot of my bed, and talking to me, and listening to me. Finally, I decided I must be going nuts and I had better try to break out of my depression or else I'd have to start taking Prozac for the rest of my life. Hence, the search began for a man (or men) to share some intimacy with me.

I certainly wasn't going to be ready for something as close as sex for at least a year, I told myself, but I needed more human contact. Some of my worst experiences happened while trying to be sociable with men my age – even my husband's friends – because they always wanted just to get me into bed. It was gross.

I read about a singles' cycling club in the local church bulletin, so I decided that would be an excellent, unpressured way to start having fun with other people. My husband and I had always been very active, and I have a lot of stamina for a gal my age. This was going to be my first outing since his death, and it seemed perfect. Our first trip was going to start near Passaic, New Jersey, and then wind through the small back-country roads for about 25 miles. A group of 30 people from 20 to 62 (me!) met at the church on our bikes at 8 am on a Saturday. We had some hot coffee and muffins together, and then got on our bikes to start the trip.

It turned out to be one of the most fun things I've ever done – but more than that, I began to go nuts over one of the guys in our group, Grant. He couldn't have been more than 35, and he had the most extraordinary build I've ever seen. Hour after hour, he pedaled ahead of me, and I couldn't stop staring at his legs. They were totally beautiful, with strong, sinewy calf muscles, and thick, sensuous thighs. He had black straight hair which stuck out in wisps from his bike helmet, and a big smile with pearly-white teeth. His mouth was enough to set me off into erotic thoughts for a whole week.

During our picnic lunch, I was able to chat with him a bit. I found out he was a volunteer church worker and was thinking of entering the priesthood someday. I thought he was one of the most delightful, sincere, young men I'd ever met, and I was totally smitten by him. I wanted to kid around with him a little so he'd remember me, and I said, "Grant, you've got the best muscles I've ever seen - you could get into the

Olympics if you change your mind about the church!" It wasn't very funny, but he laughed anyway.

I know I look pretty good for someone my age, thanks to being active and thanks to having small breasts which never did sag. My face is kind of cute when I hide my wrinkles behind sunglasses, and my pixie wash-and-wear hairstyle could suit a woman of any age. Still, Grant certainly didn't look at me with any lust in his eyes. He did notice me a bit, at least, saying, "You keep in good shape yourself, Yolanda."

The sun was burning down on us as we started the afternoon portion of our ride, and he took his shirt off, as did most of the other men. He was obviously a very athletic guy. I could see his back and shoulder muscles rippling with every turn of the pedals, and he soon was glistening with sweat.

Suddenly, I was ashamed of myself.

I realized I was daydreaming of him lying down beside me so that I could touch him, hug him, and feel him holding me. But that was always, and only could be, my husband's place. It was indecent for me to think of replacing him even in fantasy, and especially with someone I didn't know, and who was presumably a member of the church with more morals than I had.

We all had a delightful time, looking at the trees and rolling hillsides as we pedaled on, and breathing in the clean country air. Back at the church, we all agreed to meet the same time the following Saturday for another ride. That whole week, I could hardly think of anything else except *him*. Grant's image filled every inch of my imagination. I began having feelings again in my vagina which I had thought I might never have again. But they were there, for sure.

I masturbated for the first time since my husband's passing, as I daydreamed simply of touching Grant all over, and having him touch me. Even in my fantasy I wouldn't go so far as to look at or play with his manhood. I could barely wait for Saturday to arrive so I could see him again. I got rid of some of my jitters by baking a loaf of bread and an apple upside-down cake to take for everyone at lunch... I was sure that would impress him. I also went shopping for a cute biking outfit, and I settled on a pair of flared khaki shorts which made my legs look thinner than they really are, and a pretty pink T-shirt.

I was petrified he might not show up, but he did, looking just as sensational as ever. I said hi, and pretended to be merely friendly to him. I thought, *maybe he'd be flattered to know I'm having such intimate fantasies about him.* But, in reality, I knew it would probably freak him out, so of course I said nothing.

We were setting out towards a recreation area where there was a swimming pool, and several people did go swimming to cool off after the picnic lunch. Grant was one of them, and my heart beat a million times a minute as I watched him in his Speedo jumping off the diving board, and climbing out of the pool dripping wet.

I knew I had to have him – but how? I began planning something in my mind as we road our bikes back to the church.

When the ride was over, I told Grant that my husband had recently died and I wanted to donate his clothes and other possessions to the next church fund-raising rummage sale. I innocently asked him to come over Sunday night for an hour to help me take the stuff down to my car. I told him, in return, I'd cook up a nice pasta dinner for us. I was pretty surprised and pleased with myself for coming up with such a good line. How could he refuse?

Viagra, Sex, & Romance

For that night's preparations, I bought a bottle of Viagra.

I had read that some restaurant in France was sprinkling crushed-up Viagra pills into its salad dressing as a kind of aphrodisiac. I thought, *maybe this will be something to make Grant go as crazy as me – at least for one night.*

The hour approached the next night, and I carefully dissolved several of the pills into the tomato sauce. I tasted it myself, and it was impossible to tell anything had been added. Also, to make Grant feel good, I gathered some expensive stuff from my husband to donate – like golf clubs, a clock radio, and an electric shaver - so he'd think he was helping to raise lots of charity cash. I was so excited I almost developed asthma! I put on a nice, soft T-shirt and a pretty flowered skirt, and acted demure when he arrived.

We got the charity stuff into my trunk in about 15 minutes, and then I gave him a nice cold beer as I got the pasta ready. He tried to tell me not to bother, but he couldn't hide the fact that he was a little hungry, and that he knew my sauce smelled really good. So, I mildly insisted that he stay, and I think he was happy to oblige. The pasta turned out to be really good, and I gave him big dollops of the sauce. Plus, I gave him another frosty beer, and then another, as we ate. I kept peeking under the table as if I had lost something, trying to see if he was developing a hard-on. I did notice him pushing his hand down into his lap from time to time, as if something was really happening down there. One crazy thing was that I had swallowed a fair amount of the sauce too, and I think that Viagra was now making *me* feel even more horny and wild than I had been already!

Dinner was over, and I told Grant we should have some Spanish coffee in the living room. When we stood up, I noticed a definite bulge right in his crotch. My plan was working! I doubled the amount of booze in his coffee, and then set the tray down in front of us on the coffee table. We drank and chatted as we watched some news, and Grant was becoming more and more unsettled.

His penis was definitely erect now, and it was something he could no longer ignore. I asked him to turn out the room lights because of the glare on the TV screen, and when he sat back down I made a move. I started telling him what nice muscles he has, and then stroked his thigh as if I was simply kidding around with him in a playful way. But the feel of that leg in my palm made me feel sexier than I had in years. He didn't push my hand away – in fact, I felt his muscle respond and twitch under my touch, and I let my hand roam over to his erect penis. I was being so naughty but I loved it! In fact, his penis was as hard as a rock. "My," I said as I continued to stroke him and squeeze him, "you certainly do have nice muscles, Grant."

His erection was so hot in my hands, I could feel the heat right through his track suit pants. In the dark room, I slid my hand down the elastic waistband, and managed to find the tip of his penis poking right out from his underwear. It was hot and rigid, and I leaned over to put it in my mouth. I was practically drooling with desire. "No, Yolanda, no..." he said weakly as my lips settled on the crown of his cock. But he didn't resist, and I slowly slipped my mouth all the way down the shaft of his full erection, letting my saliva lubricate my tongue action. I pulled his pants down to his knees as continued sucking on his magnificent erection, licking it as if it was the world's most delightful object – which, to me, it was. He didn't touch me, he simply allowed me to suck on him and lick him until I felt his penis pulsing up inside my mouth. Thick spurts of his hot essence shot against my tongue and cheeks. I kept swallowing it all down as if it was some yummy milkshake.

I was totally satisfied to have had such a close experience with the beautiful Grant, and I kneeled down between his legs and rested my head on his lap, fully expecting him to run out at any minute. But I noticed his erection was staying totally stiff, and it still felt really hot. His hard-on just wouldn't go away. I thought, *maybe he's even getting turned on by me!*

Grant's hands began touching my face, and I thought he wanted more oral sex, so I put my mouth on his erection once again. But his hands kept roaming, and he began stroking my neck, and then he reached down into my top, under my bra, and began caressing my firm breasts. I was wondering if mine were the first breasts he'd ever touched. He must have liked them, because he kept squeezing them while I sucked his cock, and then he pulled me up onto the couch beside him. He said, "Yolanda, I don't know what we're doing, and I don't know if it's right. I've never felt this way before. It's like I'm magnetized by you." There was no way I was going to tell him it was the Viagra at work!

I let him take off my top, and then we both undressed, and he turned over onto me and slid his big, masculine, manhood into my vagina. I came within a couple of minutes, and it was one of the greatest orgasms of all time. I couldn't believe how wonderful I felt! Frankly, all thoughts of my husband, my kids, or anything else in my life before that moment were instantly forgotten. Grant kept pushing into me again and again with his long, hard erection, and he kept working it against my super-sensitive clitoris. I soon went on to have another orgasm – just as powerful as the first – before

I became exhausted with pleasure. I lay back and he continued screwing me until he climaxed for his second time. It was truly delightful to have his hot, gushing, shot of sperm inside me after being so long without it. Grant's erection finally subsided, and we lounged around for a little bit before getting dressed in the dark.

We still hadn't kissed, not even once. Even when he left shortly after, he only kissed me on the cheek. I think he was rather embarrassed or ashamed of himself, and he declined my invitations from then on. The summer and the bike trips soon ended. Now, I plan to join the cross-country ski club and the indoor tennis club for the winter. I do still miss my husband terribly, but my life can go on with nice moments of happiness. My confidence in myself is up, and I'm not afraid of being with a new man anymore. I also know that when I do meet another fine specimen, I'll be able to figure out just how to deal with him.

* * * * *

Gloria's 20th Anniversary

LOVE POTIONS CAN BE REAL - as I've found out. I'm an accountant, age 45, and my husband Bill, 53, is a city employee. Viagra has become our "love potion" and we often *both* take a pill before the special dates we plan for ourselves every couple of weeks. Viagra makes my pussy feel tingly and eager for sex, and it's pretty obvious what it does for Bill's cock. And I think it makes us feel more love for each other.

It's amazing that we've been married for 20 years, and we still feel horny as well as loving and romantic towards each other. We do have good sex without Viagra, but with it we have great sex.

On our special sexy dates we take the pills before we go out to a fancy restaurant or to a show. The best part about these evenings is the fact that our sexual heat keeps mounting higher and higher as the night progresses. By the time we get home and lock ourselves into our bedroom, we're really, really ready to make love.

One of the most memorable Viagra nights involved our 20th anniversary in July when Bill took me to a cute seafood restaurant called Isaac's right near the coast. I put on a red push-up bra so that the tops of my breasts would be exposed beneath my scoop-necked summer dress. Bill teased me, saying, "Gloria, it might get dangerous if you come out with me in that get-up..."

I realized I had chosen just the right outfit once we were at the restaurant because both Bill and our young waiter kept peeking down my dress. I guess I did look dangerous!

I sat down beside Bill so that we could both face the ocean, and because it made it easier for us to caress each other's thighs under the overhanging tablecloth. That's something we both get off on. His erection was quite developed by then, and I'd press my palm down firmly onto it when nobody was watching. He was so sensitized he lurched a bit every time I squeezed that remarkable boner of his.

As for me, I always love the feel of his hand under my dress when he strokes my thighs, and he didn't let up for a moment that night. All I had on underneath were satin panties, and I kept my legs open so that he could brush his pinky right against my pussy from time to time. I got so wet that it made me crazy. In the past, we might do that kind of under-the-table caressing for fun. But on Viagra, it was more than fun. It took on a really hot and horny aspect, almost a kind of desperation, which was great.

We started on a bottle of chilled white wine, and had a lovely dinner of poached salmon for me and swordfish with capers and lemon for Bill. Throughout it all, we kept caressing each other's thighs and genitals under the tablecloth. I think both of us could have had orgasms right then and there if we weren't careful. But we probably would have made so much noise that everyone would have stared at us! By the time we finished our main course, I think the waiter had caught on to what was happening under the table because he kept a lookout towards us from the corner of his eye. That was cute - he was getting horny too! Bill and I ordered a chocolate mousse for dessert, and it had a real aphrodisiac affect on me, as chocolate usually does. I whispered, "Bill - that's it for me. I'm ready! It's *time* to get your cock into my pussy!"

We rushed to pay the tab and get back to our car, and we began smooching and necking like teenagers right in the parking lot. I wanted to take Bill's penis in my mouth right there and suck his cock until he shot off his hot come into my mouth. But he's so romantic he wanted to make it all last longer, so he made me wait until we got home.

Bill quickly undressed himself, but he made me stop halfway. He kidded me, saying, "Gloria - don't take off your high heels or your bra no matter what happens. Otherwise I might lose my hard-on!" I laughed a little and did what he said.

I began licking him all over his body. My mouth, lips and tongue felt tremendously sensitive... and, he tasted so *good* to me. He began licking my thighs and labia with wonderful long strokes of his tongue, and I felt like I was going to climax any moment. He slowly took his mouth off my clit and turned around to face me. He pushed me onto my elbows and knees with my vagina exposed and ready behind me. My cunt felt like a warm, mushy flower just waiting to receive Bill's manly, hard cock. He mounted me doggy-style and I couldn't get enough of him.

I loved receiving his erection into me that night. He pumped it against me from behind like a pneumatic drill, and it was so wonderful I felt like I was losing my mind. Every time he slammed into me he also excited my anus and the area between my anus and cunt, sending jolts of pleasure flowing through me. From time to time, he reached around with one hand to tickle my clitoris, or reached up to squeeze my breasts, sometimes outside my bra, sometimes inside it.

Although we were both pretty close to climaxing, I told him, "Bill, please don't come yet, make it last longer, it's so good…"

We moved slowly and prolonged it for as long as we could - another 10 minutes of sliding and squeezing and caressing - and soon I was released in a wonderful gushy orgasm. I was squealing and groaning really loud as I came because it was so intense. Bill gripped my ass really tightly with his hands and controlled my movements as he neared his climax. He squeezed my cheeks so tightly it felt like his nails were digging right through my skin. But I liked it! In a couple of minutes, he began to groan and shudder behind me, and then fell forwards onto me, shooting his jism deep into me. As his wife, I felt truly fulfilled.

We napped for half an hour and then sank into a warm, leisurely, floral scented bubble bath. As luck would have it, when we went back to bed his penis was back up again like a flagpole. "Gloria, I think you are about to have the experience of a lifetime," Bill said as we started screwing all over again.

This time I got on top because Bill wanted to lie back and enjoy my rhythms. I licked his hard cock and teased him all over with my tongue. He went nuts again, which was fine with me. I shifted over and kneeled right up above his face and positioned my vagina over his mouth. He was forced to lick my clit as I rubbed it back and forth over his face, all the way from my clit down to that little sensitive area just before my asshole.

His tongue and lips on me made me get closer and closer to reaching orgasm – and the good part was that I could control the speed and intensity depending on how fast I moved and how much pressure I used to sit down on his face. I started getting close to climaxing, so I let my clit hover over his mouth as he slurped and licked at me and took me way over the edge. I couldn't control myself anymore, and I grabbed his head in both my hands and pressed his mouth hard against my cunt so that his mouth was squished hard against me. And then I came – and it was even more sensational than the first time. My juices went directly down to Bill's mouth, and I was glad about it. "Bill, does your wife taste good?" I asked him. "Do you want more? Just keep fucking me so well and I'll give you more…"

I rested there on top of him, then reached behind me and checked to see how his erection was doing. He felt as hard and eager in my hands as he did 20 years earlier on our wedding night! I grabbed his cock in my fist and squeezed it tight.

I wanted that eager cock back inside me.

I slid my pussy slowly back down over his chest hairs all the way to his cock and I started fucking him like a whore who wanted to get it over with fast. My vagina was so tingly from the Viagra and Bill's tongue job that the sensations in my cunt made my whole body shudder. Bill squeezed and caressed my breasts, and, when he ejaculated inside me, it was like fireworks going off. That was truly an anniversary to remember.

One funny thought that crosses my mind every time I think of that night was the fact that our two kids would never believe what a pair of hot and horny people their parents are… Some things are best kept secret!

* * * * *

Tarra and Mr. X

In the doctor's office, Part 1: My husband, Leo, and I are laughing politely as his doctor suggests using Viagra so we could "resume our sex lives." I guess we both wanted to pretend we were fine without having had sex at all together for more than two years. Trouble is, my husband's a heavy smoker. That, along with his high blood pressure, interfered with his vascular system and made him impotent. Now, his doctor said, with the development of Viagra, Leo would be able to achieve the extra blood flow needed to produce an erection.

But there was even more trouble.

I had been playing the part of the concerned wife all this time – but in reality I'd been screwing our neighbor in our condo complex ever since my husband developed his condition.

I was getting more turned off by my husband anyway. Leo's breath was awful from all that smoking, plus he was gaining lots of weight from not watching his sweet tooth. And, he had either forgotten or just didn't care anymore about how to make me feel loved. It was as if the day his cock stopped working, he didn't need me anymore. I knew I had to stick it out with him because of the children, but that didn't mean I had to be celibate as well.

My new guy – I'll call him Mr. X – is a fine catch who's cheating on his wife whenever he's with me. We both tell each other what wonderful mates we are, except for this one flaw of screwing each other. I've actually become quite fond of Mr. X in the past year. He's always nice to me for the short times we have together. And, he even brings me little gifts that he can hide from his wife, like a single rose, or a pair of gold earrings. I, in turn, simply revel in the luxury of being cherished by this guy.

His wife is nothing to look at. She too, like my husband, deteriorated after marriage. I don't know why some people flourish and some degenerate, but it sure does happen. Mr. X and I happened to meet because we go to the pool and spa in our condo complex, while our mates never do. I had always admired him from a distance. He looks a bit like that news announcer Peter Jennings. After we got closer, I told him about the Jennings thing, and he said he had always thought I looked like a young Barbara Walters. That made me laugh like a schoolgirl!

We met while running side by side on the treadmills late at night when all of the kids had been taken care of. We started by just talking about our day (he's a garment manufacturer and I'm a dentist) and being friendly. I liked the way he always encouraged me in my workouts. He'd say, "Tarra, your shoulders are becoming so well-defined," or, "Tarra, I can't believe you're running so much now." But the remark I liked best was when he said, "You know, Tarra, those little pools of sweat at the base of your neck can really turn a guy on..."

From time to time, if we passed each other, he'd pat my butt, or put his arm around me, or he'd massage my shoulders in an off-handed, casual way. I guess he was testing to see if I was receptive to him, and I surely was. In fact, his touches made me so turned on that I soon couldn't stand it anymore. One night, we were hot and sweaty from a 30-minute workout, and we were standing close to each other talking, and we began to kiss. It started gently, just like that. A minute later, we were clutching each other so close and hard, it was like we were screwing right through our clothing. We both knew we really needed to be together. Neither of us was actually in love with the other. We just *liked* and desired each other a lot.

What could I do? My husband had reached the bottom of his prowess and he wasn't paying any attention to me at all as a wife or woman, I let my emotions sway me. Mr. X propositioned me, and we began having sex any time and any place we could meet – about two or even three times a week. He didn't need any Viagra. He had these long, slim, erections which were the exact length I needed to be able to reach deep into my vagina and stimulate my sensitive cervix. In fact, he had everything I needed in a lover.

We'd have long, slow sex when it was possible to get to one of our offices or sneak into one of our condos when our spouses were away. If we were in my office, we'd do it right on my dentist chair, which became one of my favorite locations. The tilt of the chair makes my hips and pussy bend upwards at just the right angle for him to straddle the chair, mount me from the front, and screw me deep and hard. It's one of the most erotic experiences you can imagine if you like having deep pussy penetration.

We also had quickies on occasion right there in the athletic complex after hours when nobody was around. I could be on my back on one of weight benches, and, if it was late enough, he'd get up to lock the door and turn out the lights. Then, we'd quickly pull our gym clothes down to our knees so we could get our genitals together. Or we'd do it standing up in one of the shower stalls. It was just great sex.

I know Mr. X was also doing it with his wife from time to time, but I didn't care. I know he liked me more, and our sex acts were wonderful.

Now the big problem: my husband and I were going to have to start screwing again because of that darn Viagra – but I didn't want to give up Mr. X!

In the doctor's office, Part Two: I feel like I'm another person watching the whole scene as I nod to the urologist. I agree that it's a great idea to have Leo take Viagra so that he can make both of us happy sexually once more. And, supposedly, it would help him lead a more healthy and acive lifestyle.

But I *really* want to scream out, "damn that Viagra! I like my life the way it is! I don't want to give up Mr. X and start screwing my boring husband again!" Of course, I say nothing like that...

Leo came home the next day with his prescription, and before I had a chance to take off my pantyhose, the bastard had popped a pill. I wanted to escape and to go find Mr. X! But there was no way out. Leo was into having sex, that was for sure, and I had to be the appreciative wifey.

I said, "Leo, don't forget to brush your teeth and take a shower if you're thinking of anything, okay?" He barely did clean himself up before that stupid pill started working on his cock. He was so surprised to see his cock up in the air again, he kept looking in the mirror and staring at himself with pride. But he didn't care how the rest of him looked. Overweight, bad posture, poor skin color from the smoking. What was there to admire?

I took off my bra and the rest of my clothes, and lay down on the bed for him. Leo wasn't into pleasing me. He was into humping me for quite some time. In fact, I'd say he did it better than he ever had. After more than a year without an erection, he sure wanted some of my pussy. He couldn't wait to get his erection into me. I don't know what he thought I was doing that whole year. He must have thought that somehow my libido and vagina had put out a "Gone Fishing" sign and had closed for the season. Now, all of a sudden, he wants to have sex with me and I'm supposed to be happy about it. Actually, it felt quite nice physically, but I was so mixed up I didn't have an orgasm with Leo. Emotionally, I craved Mr. X.

After our session, I went to the athletic complex, and Mr. X was there. As always, he had that Peter Jennings look, and he let his touch linger on me whenever we passed each other. Even though I had just been laid, his gaze made my pulse race. I thought, *I can't give this up – so I won't. He's got a spouse he screw, so I can have one also.* So I never did tell Mr. X that Leo got Viagra and that we had started having sex again that very day. That was also the day I began having two lovers in my life.

Mr. X was really into me that night, and I didn't want to refuse him. Anyway, I still didn't feel sexually satisfied myself from Leo's efforts since I was just on the receiving end of it. So I figured, *why not screw Mr. X now?*

The thing I was worried about was that Mr. X would notice that I still had sperm inside me from another man, and that I'd smell different or that his penis would feel more slippery or something inside me. I didn't want Mr. X to catch on because I was scared of losing him. I had a brilliant idea - going into the whirlpool. I figured that my pussy would get cleaned out by all that swirling water. And, if my pussy felt slippery to Mr. X's cock, he'd just think it was the result of the water itself and not from sex fluids. Also, any smell I had on me from Leo would certainly disappear.

I announced that I needed to massage my aching muscles with the pressure of the hot water jets, and that Mr. X could certainly join me in the whirlpool if he wished. He didn't need a second invitation. The whirlpool was in a public area, but nobody was around. I went into the women's locker room and took off all my underwear and my tights, and just kept on my leotard as an improvised bathing suit in case someone did come in. As for Mr. X, he just used his gym shorts as a bathing suit.

I slipped into the whirlpool first, and the hot water jets really did feel wonderful on my muscles. I turned myself around and felt the jets pulsing against my pussy, cleaning out the old sperm and making me more aroused at the same time. Mr. X floated over to me from behind. Without even asking (because he knew I wanted him!) he pulled his shorts down to let his cock out, then shoved my leotard over at the crotch so he could enter my vagina without my having to undress. He began screwing me from behind in long, relaxed strokes underwater as I held onto the rim of the pool for support. It was a steamy-hot, wordless fuck and I climaxed really nicely with his cock in me and my ass bumping against him... I could feel myself coming in hot spurts, and my extra lubrication added to the mixture of both men's sperm inside me. Actually, all those juices within my vagina felt silky and luxurious. I had seen quite a lot of action that night, but I wasn't happy at all about the situation.

I didn't want two lovers, I only wanted one.

It's the fault of that damn Viagra that my husband is back in action.

Now, I have to manage the sexual attentions of two men, and it's a problem. I always have to make excuses to one or the other, and I'm constantly figuring out my schedule so I can spread out all our sex sessions. I have to give myself a break for one or two days between the two of them so my mind and my body can have a chance to get cleaned out.

It's not all that exciting for me to have two lovers, I would have been happier just having Mr. X more often. Sometimes I imagine both couples switching partners. I'd get married to Mr. X, and my Leo would get married to his wife. I know I'd be happier. It's too bad about the Viagra thing. I know I was happier before my husband found his chemical libido.

* * * * *

Viagra, Sex, & Romance

Fred and June's

Fine fishing

Adventure

VIAGRA DID WONDERS FOR ME because of a problem I've had for the past few years. When I got close to 60, I developed adult-onset diabetes, and, because of my medication, my erections never last long enough to satisfy my wife June or myself. I might be able to stick my boner inside her, but my penis would just go limp right in the middle of humping her. It was as if after the diabetes developed, something down in my balls would say 'no way, Jose' right in the middle of screwing. And then my cock would become soft and I'd lose my feelings of horniness. I've always loved the way June's vagina feels on my penis, so it was really disappointing to have to pull out my limp dick like that. I'd make June come manually because I always want to keep her happy, but I felt truly deficient.

Sometimes, I'd even dream that I was fucking June for hours like I used to do in the old days, and then I'd wake up to find my sad-looking cock just kind of hanging there.

Now, I can take Viagra whenever I want, and my cock becomes the biggest and baddest cock on the block. It's even better than it was before the diabetes problem. It's hard as a tree trunk. And it can stay stiff like that for a whole hour, which is like living a real-life dream when I've got June between my legs.

I do love screwing June. She's ten years younger than I am and she has a really beautiful ass and nice bouncy breasts. She always keeps herself pretty and smelling nice. I'm not in bad shape myself since I'm a carpenter and I'm always on the go. But, compared, to her I'm a tough old bird. And now, my cock is as tough and hard as the rest of me! I can have fun with it and screw June anyway I want. A little in the mouth, a little in the pussy. And I can lean her over our bar and fuck her from behind while we're standing up. My hard-on stays hard and her pussy stays juicy. Anything I want to do with my cock, I can. It's the greatest.

The best time we've had so far was when I took my Viagra with me for the first time during our summer vacation. June and I drove up to a camping area near Schroon Lake to do some fishing and hiking in the fresh air for a week. She came fishing with me in the mornings in our rowboat, and then we'd get back to the tent and make a nice hot lunch over the propane stove. A few of those days, in the early afternoon, I took my Viagra, and we'd lie around naked on the air mattress inside the tent and wait for the effects to begin.

Viagra, Sex, & Romance

Like clockwork, my cock always began stiffening in about 30 minutes. With June snuggling up to me on our sleeping bag, my boner would soon pop right up and she'd start sucking on it like a Popsicle.

The first afternoon made us realize how amazing our lives were going to be now that we could screw properly again. For fun, June acted like she was really scared because of my hard-on was so big and strong, and she said in a really high voice, "Oh, Fred, aren't you the big bad wolf! What a scary boner you have!" I like that kind of stuff.

Her vagina was warm and wet from the heat of the day, and I rubbed her clit in little circles the way she likes. She started breathing real heavy and her body began twitching, and that's when the real action always begins. She licked my cock all over so her saliva would make it slippery for her hand to slide up and down. It felt ten times more amazing than usual since my boner gets so hot from the Viagra.

I began teasing her by rubbing her breasts with the different fishing lures I had brought up with me. With a bunch of feathery ones, I tickled her nipples and then her clitoris as she started making little squeals of delight. Then, I took out the fake rubber worms, and wiggled them as I slowly dragged them up her body from her feet to her chest. She began moaning from the moment the rubber worms tickled her toes. The moans grew deeper as I slid the warm, rubbery mass of worms up the inside of her thighs, against the outside of her pussy, onto her clit, and then used them to tickle her lightly across her stomach and breasts. She nudged my hand down towards her cunt again and I began squishing the worms harder and harder against her widening vagina.

Meanwhile, June grabbed my cock really hard in her fist and started stroking it up and down with a strong, solid rhythm. My cock was hotter than hell and getting hotter each second. The more I played with the rubber worms in her cunt, the more horny I became as well. I actually squished three or four of the rubber worms right into her pussy and made small circles with them as I played with her clit. Her body began shuddering, and she had a wet, powerful orgasm right against my hand so that I could feel her juices and her vibrations all over my palm and fingers. June was panting out, "Yes Fred, yes Fred, yes Fred..."

That was when I decided it was my turn to fuck her. I climbed in between her legs and got my cock into her hairy little pussy and we started bouncing around on that air mattress almost like it was a trampoline. I felt like I was fucking her on an amusement park ride, bouncing up and down into her. My cock felt great and even my balls got extra hot from all that bouncy screwing action. June loved it too, and then I made her really go nuts when I grabbed a handful of those rubber worms and squished them all around in circles again on her clit. She began clutching and scratching at my back, and then came again really fast and I could feel her vagina pulsing on my hard-on.

Those extra squeezes from her cunt muscles made my cock heat up like a steam driver, and my semen burst out from my cock and into her in giant shots. It was like I was a powerful cave-man or Sasquatch or something, fucking my woman in the middle of a forest so I could shoot off my load of come into her. I didn't care if the power I felt was coming from the Viagra pill or not – I felt like the manliest man in the state.

Our fishing trip still wasn't over. On another day, we went out in the motorboat after I had taken my lunchtime Viagra, and, we lazed around in the boat having a smoke and

Viagra, Sex, & Romance

dangling our lines in the lake. Before we knew it, right in the middle of the lake I developed another one of my big hard-ons and it was practically poking right out of my bathing suit. June said, "I think that boner needs some fresh mountain air," and pulled my pants down to expose it completely. Then she added, "Fred, I think it needs some exercise" as she began stroking it hard with her hand.

Although there were other boats in the area, none were close enough to see what we were up to. June kneeled down and started sucking on my hard-on, using her amazing tongue action to lick the top as she sucked on me. The boat was rocking a bit, and it got really tipsy, but we didn't care – it was all just too much fun. I said, "June, I think that pussy of yours is calling out to me because it needs some fresh air too."

June slipped off the bottom half of her bikini, and her bright white tan line made her cunt and ass look really white and bright and fuckable. It was like making a target for me to hit with my cock. I thought the boat was too wobbly for her to lie on her back, so I kneeled down and got her to turn around and point her creamy white ass at my cock.

I slid right into her cunt from behind, hugging her tightly around the waist so that we wouldn't jiggle around too much and tip the boat right over. Out in nature I liked being uncivilized, and as I fucked her back-asswards I was grunting and groveling like an ape, pawing her breasts and clit, and biting the back of her neck. I came in big bursts of semen, gripping her beautiful ass in my hands to bring her cunt into me as deeply as I could. After I was finished, June said she had started feeling a little seasick so she wasn't going to have a climax herself. She added that I could owe her one, and I said that was fine with me.

Viagra, Sex, & Romance

We actually did screw in the forest on our last day, right out in the open. I had taken my blue pill at lunchtime as usual, and we decided to take a hike on the nature trail, and I became friskier and friskier. June thought it was cute the way my hard-on was bulging in my pants, and when we sat down to rest on one of the hills, she stroked my penis under my shorts. That was enough for me to get started!

We were on an exposed trail where everyone could have seen us, so I took her by the hand until we found a little secret area. It was a hidden little cave formed from big boulders where we could look out at the trail, but nobody could see in. June was into it as much as I was, and her pussy was already nice and warm and moist from the heat of the day. The cave was really tiny, so I lay down on the earth and let her get on top of me. This time she swivelled herself around so that I was looking at her back and her ass as her cunt went up and down on my cock. I reached up to touch her bouncing breasts and let her nipples rub against my palms as she moved. She played with her clit and my balls with her hands as she was screwing me, and we both I got really steamy. I was barely able to stall myself from climaxing before she came. As soon as she did, I climaxed too, and my come began shooting out of my cock like a geyser.

When we got back to the city, we decreased our screwing activity down to more normal levels, but we both think that was one of the best vacations we've ever had.

One thing I can say is that shoving my new-found hard-ons into her pussy is still as great or even better than it was before I developed diabetes, and I have medical science to thank for that.

* * * * *

Valerie's Double Header

I'M A 19-YEAR-OLD CO-ED at NYU and I never had a very high sex drive. Guys hit on me because I look pretty (they say I look like Chelsea Clinton but with bigger boobs), and because I'm comfortable talking and joking around with them. Guys don't intimidate me. I grew up with three brothers, so I always had to be a little tough to make sure they wouldn't bully me. For me, going out with a guy is like a fun, romantic thing to do. But it's not the kind of thing that makes me yearn for him to lick my pussy or for me to desire to fondle his penis.

My last boyfriend was really cute and I liked him a lot. Most of the time when we had sex together it hardly did anything for me. I kind of pretended that it was erotic, but I'd end up daydreaming of totally different things while he was pushing his penis into my vagina. He didn't even seem to notice! I was even wondering if my girlfriends were lying when they'd talk about how good sex feels. I do masturbate once in awhile and I get nice little orgasms, but there's nothing so wonderful about it. Then, last summer, when the women's magazines began running articles about Viagra and how it worked wonders on women, I decided I'd give it a try to see if it made me and my vagina feel any different. I really didn't think much would happen.

Big surprise!

The pills were very easy to buy in New York. One pharmacy actually had prescriptions that were signed in advance by a doctor, and they just filled in a name and sold me a bottle. I planned to take my first pill when there'd be a guy around to screw, and I tried to figure out who the lucky guy should be.

I picked Aaron, a fellow law student, to be my first Viagra "screwee", if that's the right word. I'd hardly call him my lover because I was just using him for one thing. He was part of my experiment. He was a hunky kind of guy, about 5'10", with a great physique and a face like Matt Damon's. We met at the first summer job for both of us in a big downtown law firm. For both of us, it was intimidating to work with such important lawyers for the first time, so being in the same boat made us develop a bond.

Aaron and I bought weekend time-shares in the same Hamptons house for the summer, and we drove up together when beach season began. All the other people in the house were into partying and boozing, and we tagged along with them at night when they went to the local bars. Like most of the guys, Aaron would talk to quite a few girls at the bar, but he never scored. As for the girls, they seem to like flirting as a means to boost their egos or to show off to their girlfriends about how they could attract guys. I figured Aaron would be ripe for the picking.

I took my first Viagra pill just before going to one of those bars on a Friday night with Aaron and the rest of the gang from our house. I also carefully put a strip of three condoms in my pocket just in case the pill really would work for me. I didn't tell anybody I had taken the pill, not even Aaron. There was a live band playing and we drank a few beers and hung around as usual. I was waiting to see if I would feel anything new down in my vaginal area. I flirted with some of the good-looking guys there, but, as usual, that didn't make me feel turned on.

But within an hour, I really did start to feel excited. It was quite amazing to feel that I was beginning to get special signals from my vagina and clitoris. I was excited and tingly in that area, and I actually wanted to touch myself because I was sure it would feel really, really good. I was getting horny! A lot of the guys in the bar seemed really attractive, and I almost found myself picking up a stranger instead of Aaron. There sure were a lot of handsome, horny guys everywhere. Any one of them would have wanted me to suck their cocks or would have wanted to suck on my vagina. I know what teenage guys are like. But I didn't want to do it with a stranger that first time on Viagra because I probably wouldn't have felt comfortable. And I wanted to enjoy the experience as much as possible.

Viagra, Sex, & Romance

The band started playing *You're the One that I Want* and everyone began jumping around and screaming out the words. I asked Aaron to dance. It was really sweaty and hot in there, and everyone was going wild and bumping into each other in time to the music. They played that song forever, I think because they didn't know too many songs, and then they switched to that old slow song, *Blue Bayou*. People pulled their partners really close, and began dirty dancing. I took Aaron in my arms for the first time, and it felt pretty good to have his muscular chest pressing against my breasts... and that was when IT happened.

My vagina really went ballistic. It began to feel like it was glowing in a way I had never felt before. I hugged Aaron closer so that his thigh rubbed against my crotch, and I could clearly feel my clit becoming hotter and more excited as he rubbed against me. It was the first time became so excited from sexual feelings in my vagina. As we continued dancing, I could feel Aaron putting the moves on me, stroking my back and hair, and hugging me close to make sure my breasts kept rubbing against him. He must have thought this was going to be his lucky night – and he was right. It didn't take a genius to realize he was getting a big hard boner himself. I could feel it clearly pressing against my leg, sort of like the way a horny dog does it to you when you're sitting around. I knew he'd be ready to have some fast sex, which is what I wanted that night.

By the time that long slow song ended, he was putting his mouth on top of mine to try to give me a kiss. Even my mouth felt more susceptible to erotic stimulation, so I kissed him back, and the sensation of our tongues sliding and twisting around together was really hot. I was ready to start my experiment with my vagina and my mouth, to try and feel if I was going to have some wonderful sex now that the Viagra was having its effect on me.

The other kids from our house thought it was strange that Aaron and I were becoming so close. Usually they say you shouldn't screw anyone from your summer house because it becomes so uncomfortable if you split. But I wasn't thinking so logically. I was thinking with my clit, not my brain.

We both had a couple of peach schnapps shooters and we decided to go out for a stroll along the beach. Aaron had his arm around my shoulders and he said, "Valerie, I feel so good being with you, I'm starting to get feelings for you..."

That made me feel uneasy because I didn't want to get into a whole relationship thing with him. I told him he didn't have to say anything, and I think he got the message. We were soon standing around on the grassy area just before the sand. In the distance, shimmering black waves washed into shore. The sky was so dark and clear, and the stars were sparkling like diamonds above us. A perfect night to get laid!

Aaron started the usual guy stuff of kissing me on the neck and so on, and then touching my breasts on the outside of my T-shirt before going under my shirt to undo my bra. In the past I'd just play along with my boyfriends and pretend it felt really good - but that night was the first time my whole body really did feel fantastic. We sat on the grass, and Aaron lifted up my shirt so that he could lick my nipples, and it was the most delicious feeling my breasts have ever had. I pulled his head harder against me, and he obligingly rubbed his wet tongue around both of my breasts, and nibbled on my nipples. I admit I wasn't really reciprocating, because I was just lying back and enjoying everything too much to care. But Aaron was obviously enjoying it too, so it seemed fine.

Viagra, Sex, & Romance

When he began fondling my vagina through my jeans I almost went wild. I thought, *so this is what the other women are talking about when they say sex feels so wonderful.* I wanted him to keep on stroking my pussy forever, but more than that I wanted him to finger me directly on my clit and vulva. He was taking the longest time to undo my jeans so I just undid them myself and he stuck his hand right down into my panties onto my naked vagina. My pussy was getting really wet the more he fingered me and I began to breathe faster. I was thinking about how great his mouth felt on mine, and how much nicer it would feel to have his mouth and tongue right on my vagina – and how nice my mouth would feel to have an eager cock inside it.

I swivelled around so that my pussy would be near his mouth, and he obligingly started to do me. He quickly pulled my jeans all the way off so he could get his face right into my crotch. I spread my legs wide, and grabbed the hair on the back of his head so I could push him down harder onto my pussy. He started by licking the inside of my thigh, and then slid his tongue right across my vagina to the other thigh. I was really going crazy and I was happy because my pussy was feeling such a high intensity of arousal. I almost couldn't stand getting so much pleasure. I wanted him to lick me and suck on my pussy and make me have one orgasm after another. I admit I was grabbing his hair really tightly, and I began forcefully pushing my vagina at his mouth.

I still hadn't touched him, but I could feel his hips humping up and down near my head, and I suddenly wanted to start playing with his penis. I undid his belt and zipper and reached in to free his boner. He was hot, and the smell of his aftershave aroused me. It made me want to suck on his cock. I began licking the top of it, flicking my tongue on the tiny opening, and sliding my mouth and lips around the sides as deeply as I could. He was trying to jam his hard-on as deeply into my mouth as he possibly could, and I was still pushing his head harder into my vagina. I was hugging his head between my thighs, and I felt like I could have kept going in that 69 position all night!

I was getting really close to climaxing and I felt I was losing control for the first time in my life. I had to stop sucking on his cock right away because I was afraid I'd bite down on it really hard and hurt him badly when I actually started coming. So, I lay on my back with my knees spread out and held his head with both my hands, moving his mouth exactly to where I wanted his tongue to lick me.

I made him go in nice, long, hard strokes from the bottom of my pussy to my clit and back. All of a sudden my clit went nuts, and I held his head right on top of it as my hips began convulsing like I was having an epileptic fit. I climaxed right into his mouth with the most amazing orgasm I have ever experienced. It was like my pussy itself felt happy and fulfilled for showing me what heights of pleasure it was capable of feeling. I think I found out what I had been missing for so many years.

Aaron was still in the 69 position and I was still gripping his head with both my hands at my crotch level and I looked down to see him peering up at me. "Aaron, you're amazing – you made me have the greatest orgasm I've ever had," I said. That remark, unfortunately, turned out later to have been a big mistake! I didn't realize it then, but this guy who was having such a close encounter with my wet pussy was starting to fall in love with me!

He said, "It's funny, but when you came it really turned me on too, Val."

Anyway, his big boner was still facing my mouth and I wanted to see how it would feel inside my pussy. I pulled out a condom and unravelled it onto his cock, then turned him around into the missionary position so that his cock was pointing into my vagina. I said, "Do me, Aaron, do me, I really want you inside me."

He stuck his hard penis deeper and deeper into my pussy. *Yes*, I thought, *yes, this is what fucking is all about. My vagina feels so wonderful.* Aaron was very athletic, so he was pounding his cock quite heavily against my labia and into the interior of my vagina, and every part of my female organ appreciated his manhood. He kept saying my name, "Valerie, Valerie, Valerie."

I almost came again, but he got himself into a bit of a rush and he started going double-speed, ramming his erection into me. He soon started shaking and grunting, and having his own orgasm. It had been an excellent experience for me, and it seemed excellent for him too. After a couple of minutes, he took off the condom and dumped it in the sand, and we walked back to the bar in a really good mood.

By then it was midnight, and the place was really hopping and everybody was squeezed in butt to butt, dancing in time to the music. It seemed like the crowd had become one single mass of people, all gyrating up and down in unison to that old Rolling Stones song *It's Alright*. The smell of deodorant, perfume and cigarette smoke hung in the air like a dense fog, and it made the room seem full of sex. Aaron and I squeezed in to dance with the crowd.

A really cute guy who looked like Tom Cruise kept bumping into me - even though I was dancing with Aaron and he was dancing with another girl. For some strange reason we kept looking at each other, and he'd brush his arm against my back when nobody was noticing. For a moment he actually placed his palm on the small of my back. I thought that was very forward of him, but I really liked it. I was getting turned on all over again. There was a super-strong attraction between us. My heart started beating quickly whenever I felt his touch or caught his eye.

Aaron took a bathroom break, and the new guy's girl left him and sat down. The band started playing *No Woman, No Cry,* and he boldly came up to me and asked me to dance. I was going crazy. I took his hand as he led me onto the floor, and we held each other tight. I didn't even know his name, nor did he know mine. The Viagra must have started a chain reaction within my sex organs and I couldn't turn it off. My vagina was ready for some new action right away. I felt an urgency in my clitoris, and I pressed it against him while we danced. I could feel his hard-on growing behind his zipper, grinding against my clit. At chest level, he must have been able to feel my heart beating against him. We were dancing in a thick pack of kids and the lights were low and, luckily, Aaron wasn't in sight.

The new guy's left hand roamed from the back of my t-shirt to my side, and he slyly began caressing my right breast with his outstretched thumb. I didn't stop him. In fact, I held him closer. I felt like such a slut. His thumb was squirming out, reaching all the way up to my nipple, and then rubbing it. I was so turned on and it felt so wonderful. I wanted him to just rub my breasts all over, and to caress my vagina and make it even hotter than it was. It was like vertical foreplay.

Aaron had returned and he was hovering at the bar talking to some of the kids from our summer share. He didn't seem too happy about my being with another guy, but at least he couldn't see the guy was touching my breasts. In any case, I never told Aaron I wanted to go out with him or anything. The new guy finally told me his name was Bruce and he asked me if I wanted to go for a walk, so I quickly left with him.

I wasn't planning to be too intimate with the new guy. I mean, I just got laid an hour earlier. But before I knew it, we were out walking along a secluded area of shoreline and he put his face in front of mine to kiss me. I was curious about how it would feel to kiss him, so I did. We could see and hear the waves crashing and it was all quite beautiful. We truly did have an animal attraction for each other, and when you add that onto the Viagra chain reaction bubbling within me, I became putty in Bruce's hands.

Bruce felt totally different to me than Aaron - much more passionate and powerful, and more in tune with my feelings. We lay down on the sand, and he pulled up my T-shirt without even asking, and began massaging my breasts. It felt even better than when we had been dancing. I was so relieved to finally feel him touching me that I only briefly resisted. He was soon licking my nipples, and he was as wonderful as I had imagined he'd be. The funny things was, he was licking me right where Aaron's dried up saliva must have been and he never noticed. Bruce reached down into my pants and inserted his finger deep into my vagina, with his palm resting against my clit, and he slowly began massaging his hand and the inserted finger around in circles on my vagina. He could sense I was going to come and that I was particularly vulnerable to suggestion, so he pulled his jeans down to his knees, exposing his erection as he wanted to fuck me right then and there.

Bruce's penis was much bigger than Aaron's and much hotter. I licked the tip briefly just to taste it, and it almost filled up my mouth. I was craving for him to push it into my pussy.

Viagra, Sex, & Romance

Luckily I had another condom on me! I gave it to him, and he laughed and said, "You're almost as fast as me." He rolled it onto his erection, and he instantaneously began screwing me. He knew what he wanted, and what I wanted. I was getting more cock action that night than I had experienced in years, and I really liked it. I loved the feeling of his big boner in me, and feeling him squeeze my breasts hard with his hands. Both of us had fantastic orgasms in a simultaneous burst of energy just two minutes after we started screwing. I don't think we said even a single word to each other during the time we walked back to the club. It was all just animalistic feelings.

That was my Viagra night, and I'm not proud of it.

I really was a slut and I blame it on that pill.

Bruce never called me, and, although I never told Aaron that I went all the way with Bruce, he was pretty hurt about my leaving him at the bar. Then, for some strange reason, Aaron started thinking he was in love with me, and he began sending me flowers and little love notes in some kind of manly attempt to win my affections. But I was never in love with him to begin with. Plus, I don't like having guys being infatuated with me, so I've been having to make lots of excuses. It's been a little hard on me, working with him in the same office.

But I definitely would do it all again.

* * * * *

Viagra, Sex, & Romance

Ethan

and the

Spice Girls

A SPICE GIRLS FANTASY WEEK sure sounded good to me. I may be an old guy at 67, but so what? I'm still pretty good at having sex, and with Viagra I'm *really* great at it. Viagra and my special women friends helped me fulfil my Spice Girls fantasy. Those Spice Girls are the sexiest and most beautiful performers I have ever laid my eyes on. Every time I see them on TV my cock starts to pick up and my pulse races like crazy. My dream was to screw each one of them on a different night, and I got five of my gals to help me do it – or at least pretend to do.

I like having regular sex with several women friends instead of having just one girlfriend. I've met some of them at our neighborhood country and western bar, and a couple of others are "working" girls from a strip bar I go to every week.

Viagra, Sex, & Romance

None of us are too serious with each other, and that's the way we like it. I was already married for 30 years until my wife passed away, so I had enough of that wifey stuff, you know, "Ethan, you should do this, and Ethan, you should do that."

I take turns going on dates with my women so nothing ever gets too close or sticky with any of them. That's what keeps our relationships lively. We have a rule, 'ask me no questions and I'll tell you no lies.' I see them when I want and how I want. And usually, the way I want to see them is all dolled up in pretty outfits and with nice feminine make-up on. That makes it all the more fun when I take the clothes off them!

Don't get me wrong. I am a gentleman. I always pay for dinners and movies and so on. I even take my dates shopping and buy them shoes and dresses. I'm a retired diesel mechanic with a good pension, so I've got the time and money for it. I'm not hard on the eyes either - I'm 5'10", only a little bald, and muscular in a stocky kind of way. And I'm always very polite to any woman. I keep them happy and they keep me happy. I think I'm allowed to follow my wishes and desires. A woman who goes with me has the right to decide if it suits her or not. If so – fine. If not, I hope she finds someone else who suits her better.

My wonderful Spice Girls fantasy week was pretty simple to set up, and it turned out to be even more fun than I had ever hoped for. All the action was planned for my den, where I have a big screen TV wired to a super sound system. I had planned to play Spice Girls music videos and the Spice Girls movie during our love-making. And, for extra atmosphere, I put a bunch of Spice Girls posters up on the walls. I also set up a foam mattress in front of the screen for us to bounce around on, and I covered it with a nice purple satin sheet.

The first step was to line up my dates and ask each of them to dress up like one of the Spice Girls for our special night. It didn't take much convincing, because they thought it would be fun to play-act like that. And, to make the deal sweeter, I bought the outfits each woman needed - like a teenie-tight bare-midriff black pant suit for Scary, a leopard skin leotard for Posh, baby-doll pj's for Baby, a see-through lace bra for Sporty, and a bustier and miniskirt for Ginger. And, I got some of those Spice Girls tattoos, the ones that you stick on with water, and I told the women to put one on each breast. In the end, one of my gals didn't like the whole idea, so I had my best girlfriend Sherry play two parts, both Ginger and Baby, on different nights, because she was the one who was most excited about the idea.

Saturday night arrived, and I was ready to rock and roll with my first Spice Girl date.

Sherry - who was going to act as Baby - came that night dressed in the baby-doll pj's, and we had a couple of cocktails as a Spice Girls video played in the background. Sherry said, "Ethan, you're nuts - but you're nuts in a fun kind of way." Actually, I think *she's* more nuts than I am!

I took one of my Viagra pills to be extra sure that we'd be able to suck and fuck for a real long time. Sherry got a bit loaded, and started swaying to the music and then dancing and prancing like Baby Spice does as she really got into it. It was really cute and sexy. She began singing along, and then yelling out "Girl Power!" with a British accent, which was really funny. I had planned to start undressing "my" Spice Girls about half-way through the video presentation. But I couldn't wait that long!

Viagra, Sex, & Romance

My boner got so hot from having my own live Spice Girl dancing for me that I hopped down on my knees onto the satin sheets and began licking her cunt right through the baby dolls as she gyrated in my face. I kept my eyes wide open to be able to watch the TV, and it was easy for me to pretend that my Baby Spice was the real thing. When she began peeling off the bottoms, my boner almost went straight up in the air. Man, I love that Viagra.

She teased me for half an hour as the video played, shaking my cock in her hands and kissing it up and down, and brushing her hair all over my body from my ass to my shoulders. The great thing is that all of her motions, especially when she played with my cock, were in time to the music. I did a lot of finger action inside her and around the soft lips of her vagina, always in time to the music. My hard-on stayed hard forever, and I knew that I was headed for a fantastic ejaculation. I took off Sherry's top, and licked her breasts with the Spice Girls tattoos on them, and told her, "Baby Spice, I love you Baby," while she sang along to the choruses.

She was saying, "Oh Ethan, Baby Spice needs you too," as I pushed my boner into my Baby Spice's cunt. I was telling myself, *even the real Baby Spice couldn't feel better than this – I must be a genius!*

Sherry started to come before I did, I think because of all the advance finger action, and as she came she yelled out "Girl Power! Girl Power!" That was enough for me to go nuts, and I orgasmed right deep into my Baby Spice's vagina. It was like a dream come true.

We both lay there panting until we caught our breath, and Sherry told me she couldn't wait until the end of the week when she'd become Ginger Spice.

The funny thing was that Sherry's great act made me even more fond of her, and I almost wanted her to try to be all the Spice Girls. But I went on to the other three anyway with varying degrees of success. I did take my Viagra and I did get hard and have a great orgasm into each of their pussies each night, but the other three didn't get into it as much as Sherry did.

Sporty was pretty good, and she copied a whole bunch of the group's jumping moves which made her pussy the hottest of all. When I put my hard-on into her hot, juiced-up vagina I felt like she was squirting all over! I rubbed Sporty's steamy clit with my fingers while my cock was inside her, and my hand got drenched. She was so heated up she came fast, and I came almost right away after her. That part was excllent.

Posh was exquisite in her leopard skin outfit, but she got too drunk to dance much, so I just fucked her from behind as she lay there, mainly because my cock was so hard and I needed to come. Scary was black and beautiful, but she wasn't into acting much, so she wasn't all that much fun. Still, she had great legs and the tattoo on her breast looked really nice against her black skin. We just screwed in the missionary position and she left with a little kiss good-night.

The last night, though, Sherry returned and put on the greatest Ginger show ever. She even colored her hair in streaks to match Ginger's, and she went wild when I turned up the music video. But this time, when I got crazy to fuck her she said, "Not so fast, lover. If you really want me, you have to show me." She decided she was going to tie me up and make me beg before we did anything else. I was so horny I had to agree. She took a belt and tied my hands in front of me, and pushed me down on my knees on the mattress. Then she pulled up a barstool and demanded, "Now, Ethan, let's see you beg if you want Ginger Spice that much."

I figured I'd play along, so I said, "Ginger Spice, I love you, I need you to suck me and fuck me! Please Ginger!"

She said, "Maybe, Ethan, maybe. But first you need to pray, and you need to pray really well." She took off her tights, and spread her naked legs apart as she sat above me in her bustier. "Pray," she said, "you made me dress up to be the object of your desires, now pray to receive your gift."

I answered, "Yes Ginger Spice, I'll pray, I'll pray!" So I licked her clit and stuck my tongue into her perfumed cunt until she came all over my mouth.

She said, "Now I'll teach you a lesson you need to learn for running around with other women!" She turned me over onto my back, then took the belt of a bathrobe and tied my hands to the table legs behind me. I was totally under my Spice Girl's "Girl Power" now. I had no idea what to expect. I was pretty sure she wouldn't hurt me - but she did cause me to get blue balls.

Ginger began lightly caressing my cock with small movements of her hand and fingers, teasing me so that I became more and more horny without coming. The, she knelt over me and rubbed her moist vagina on my cock, still refusing to let me enter her.

My erection was almost bursting from the effects of the Viagra, and it began to hurt. I needed release! I began pleading with her: "Please, Ginger, please, make me come! I can't stand this anymore! Lick me or fuck me, but just make me come!" Still, she had other ideas. She moved her tattooed breasts to my mouth and made me suck on her nipples as she kept on teasing me by tickling my balls. The pain in my penis was becoming very unpleasant, and was much worse than ordinary blue balls since it affected my balls and my cock. "Not so fast, Ethan, not so fast..." she said. I was totally at her mercy.

After I pleaded and begged for another ten minutes, she finally slipped her vagina down onto my erection as I lay there defenseless with my hands tied. I tried to move my cock quickly inside her so I could come, but whenever I did, she lifted herself up and off my erection, leaving me high and dry and in pain. I really needed to have an orgasm. I began telling her that she was the best Spice Girl in the world, and she made me more crazy than any other woman I knew - and the funny thing about it was that I meant it.

Finally, my Ginger said, "Now, you deserve to come." She started moving her cunt more rapidly with every compliment I gave her. This time she didn't tease, and both of us came almost at the same time. For me, having the release through my orgasm after waiting so long and needing it so desperately made the climax feel like I was riding a Roman candle on the Fourth of July.

A little later, after she untied me and we were lying around, she stayed in her Ginger persona and made up a whole long funny story about how she had to leave the group so she could follow her own destiny to become a big solo star. I laughed through it all, and I told her she already was a big star in my eyes, and I really meant it. My Sherry/Ginger was the perfect topping to my Spice Girls week.

I know I've always loved Sherry's sense of humor and the way she can play-act. She sort of outdoes me. I was happy when she slept over that night. And, we do actually hang around together a lot. I know she's a threat to my new way of life, but the glamor of my way of life does seem to fade from time to time. I'll keep you posted!

* * * * *

FULL SPECTRUM ENZYMES™

Pure Plant Source Enzymes

Full Activity Level pH2 to pH12

Our body receives enzymes from two sources, those it makes and those that it gets from the food we consume. Enzymes occurring in foods aid in the digestion process so our body's enzymes do not have to do all the work. Enzymes play an important role in the proper digestion of the food we eat.

Enzymes are the essential catalysts that makes metabolism possible.

Poor eating habits and the low enzyme content of highly processed food greatly diminishes our enzyme supply. Over heating of foods will drastically reduce the enzyme content. Enzyme depleted foods rob the body of its enzyme potential. Aging is another factor that can reduce the body's ability to produce sufficient enzymes for optimum digestion.

ORGANIKA's Full Spectrum Enzymes™ is a professional formulated plant source base digestive enzyme complex that has been used by many individuals as a digestive aid. It is specifically used for the digestion of Proteins, Cellulose, Carbohydrates ,fats and sugars under a wide range of ph levels within our digestive system (pH2-pH12).

The digestion of enzyme deficient food is an extremely energy-consuming task for our body's metabolism to handle .... For some individuals **Full Spectrum Enzymes™** may be a means to overcome some of the gastrointestinal problems associated with poor eating habits or incorrectly prepared foods.

ORGANIKA'
Your Canadian Choice ▮✦▮

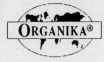

ORGANIKA®

ORGANIKA HEALTH PRODUCTS INC.
Richmond, BC, Canada V6V 2H9

© 08/93

Samantha, Viagra,

and the

Therapist

I'M A WORKING WIFE with three kids and no time or energy for sex. Viagra can't change that. But the combination of Viagra and counseling really helped me and my marriage.

Dennis and I were married almost ten years ago when he was 31 and I was 34. Our marriage had deteriorated since then because he was never very good at being a husband. He'd rarely help with the kids or the housework, so it meant I was busy 24 hours a day. I had to keep up my job as a bookkeeper, plus do all the housework, help the kids with their homework, get everyone's clothes washed and ready, and all the rest of it. So things went downhill.

There's just so much I can do in a day, and having long, drawn-out sex with my husband isn't one of them. That's the bottom line. If he wanted some sex, fine. I liked it enough to go along with him for a little while. He's always had a really thick cock (about double any other man's that I've seen), and that's a turn-on for me. I was happy it wasn't twice as long too - I think that would have killed me.

At the beginning of our relationship, I was crazy about having sex with him. It was a thrill to have him trying to force that thick erection in through the lips of my vagina. We were always very spontaneous, and he had a lot of hard-ons. I loved going to drive-ins with him and getting into the back seat and screwing. And, because my vagina opened up a little wider when I was on my hands and knees, I loved it when he'd mount me and pump from behind. His thick, short boner was the perfect size for doggy-style intercourse.

But, as the years went by I started to lose interest in sex and I just wanted him to get it over with as quickly as possible. I'd be happy if he'd ejaculate fast into my vagina and then pull out and let me sleep. The emotional and horny parts of my heart used to get excited when we'd get physical – but those days were obviously gone.

He said I was becoming frigid, but the real point was that I just didn't want to be sexy with *him*. We were arguing all the time. I told him, "Dennis, if you want me to be sexy, you have to help me. You do the vacuuming and send your kids to have their baths, and meanwhile I'll lounge around a little and start to feel sexy."

His excuse was, "But Samantha, I work all day too." So, once in blue moon he'd help. But usually he'd just flop down in front of the TV until his horniness went away. *My* idea of an aphrodisiac would have been to watch him scrubbing the sink or bathtub with Comet! Meanwhile, he had been reading about women getting horny from taking Viagra, and he thought that would be the quick solution to cure "my" problem of becoming more frigid each year.

I told him even if Viagra worked I didn't want to become more horny anyway, because who would be taking care of all the household problems while we're screwing around with each other? His answer was, "Samantha, there's obviously something wrong with you." What a guy thing to say.

Then we went for counseling – and that, along with the Viagra, really made a difference in our lives.

Going to the therapist was the best thing we ever did. He noted that I had a lot of repressed anger (no kidding!) all these years because of the way Dennis was acting. And, he said I was also repressing my own pleasure and becoming frigid because I didn't want to please Dennis. Meanwhile, since Dennis is the lazy son-of-a-gun that he is, nothing was ever going to change him. During therapy it became clear that we would likely have ended up divorcing sooner or later. The idea of divorce was such a drag that we both decided to make a real effort to find a solution.

Presto! The therapist came up with a few ideas. He told Dennis that it was up to him to find a way to make me happy, because that's part of his job as being half in charge of the household. They talked for a few minutes – then Dennis, who's normally a pretty cheap guy except when it comes to his cars or golf, agreed to pay for a housecleaner for a whole day each week. And, he agreed to take charge of putting the kids to bed one night a week. The therapist figured that I'd start feeling less pressured about everything, and that would be a big step towards solving our sexual problem. I liked the whole concept so much I told Dennis I'd even try using Viagra if the time was right.

Our new housecleaner really took over a big part of my work, and my night off from the kids was great for me. So, after the first two weeks I began to feel more free than I had in years. And, I felt warm inside because it showed me that Dennis really did care enough about me to pay for the cleaner. I was able to look at him fondly and start to like him again, and to think of having real sex with him again.

One Sunday morning when the kids left early, he began kissing me and I really responded. It felt a lot like the old days before we had kids, when I enjoyed squeezing his extra-thick erection in my hands while I licked the tip. I liked the fact that I could barely get my mouth around it. I had almost forgotten how excited it used to make me. It seemed like years since we had wild and crazy sex. I realized Dennis was partly right in saying I was becoming frigid, even though it *was* his fault. Anyway, that Sunday when we re-launched our sex life, I did want our love-making to last longer than the quickies we had been having.

I turned around on our bed and let him do cunnilingus on me while I sucked his cock and put his balls in my mouth one at a time. He was surprised and happy to have me paying attention to him again, and he really sucked my clit well and licked my vagina all over to turn me on too. My juices were flowing, and I felt great. He squeezed his thick boner into me and began fucking me, but that didn't make me have an orgasm as it used to. I had to finger my clit and make myself come. It was nice, but no cigar, and even Dennis noticed there were no skyrockets in flight. It seemed like I really did need something to kick-start my sexuality again, and I figured maybe Viagra could do the trick.

Dennis brought some home for me, and I took a pill the next Saturday night as we were about to go out on a date without the kids. He was pretty pleased with himself for coming up with the idea, and he even arranged for a baby sitter. Dennis was really starting to score points with me! I got a bit dressed up in a skirt and a girly-looking top.

For fun, we figured we'd take the van out to a drive-in because we hadn't been to one in years. Titanic was playing, and I thought the romantic aspects of it would help us get into the right mood for making love later. But even as we were driving past the suburbs to the movie, the Viagra started making my vagina feel extra tingly. There wasn't going to be a "later" because I was needing it now.

My clitoris quickly became the focus of my attention because it felt like there was energy radiating from it all the way down my newly sensitive thighs. I took Dennis' hand off the steering wheel and put it on the inside of my thigh where he could feel the warmth of my crotch, and he quickly got the message. He caressed my thighs, saying, "You sure have the greatest legs in the world, Samantha - I could touch them forever." But I wanted him to stroke my pussy. I wanted him to touch me there, and to touch me a lot.

I settled forward in the seat so I could spread my legs more, and his fingers quickly found their way in through the crotch of my panties and to my vagina. His hand began massaging my bush and tickling my clit and rubbing deeply against vulva. I was so horny it was amazing! My heart was pounding extra-fast within me as my expectations of reaching a tremendous climax rose. I spread my legs out wider, and I began panting as his manipulations brought me closer to exploding. I wanted him to touch me like that forever – or for at least an hour! – because of the great vibrations that were rushing through me.

Viagra, Sex, & Romance

I need to touch his cock, and I reached over to his lap and felt it hard and hot, and I undid his zipper and belt. I didn't want him to drive off the road, so I was careful not to make him climax. But I did what he used to always like – I ran my nails around the tip of his dick, and then slid them up and down, hard enough to let him feel the sharpness, but not hard enough to scratch him. He began squirming in his seat while his right hand continued probing into my pussy with a new eagerness. His middle finger found my G-spot and he started massaging it in little circles. I could feel that area inside my vagina becoming erect and sensitive, and just before we had to turn off the road to the drive-in, I came in hot, fast, delicious spurts. It had been years since I felt so sexy, and I was happy about it. The funny thing was, I was still horny.

Dennis laughed a little as he paid for our tickets when we drove past the booths. "You sure don't seem frigid anymore, Sweetie. I think you're going to be a great drive-in date tonight," he said.

I joked back, "Well, Dennis, let's see if you're going to be a good drive-in date. Let's park way off in the back corner where nobody can see us…" Denis pretended to be *really* shocked, and he made a funny expression by raising his bushy eyebrows. And he did drive off to the most secluded area.

We didn't see much of the movie that night! As soon as the credits began rolling, we locked up the doors and skedaddled down to the back of the van and pulled off everything we were wearing from the waist down. I kneeled down beside him, stretched my mouth around his thick boner and gave him some of the best head he's ever had. My goal was to get that big erection into my pussy because I was aching for that feeling of stretching and penetration.

It was years since I appreciated the size of his erection as much as I did that night. My pussy was really wet from having that first orgasm while we were driving and the effects of the Viagra still hadn't worn off. So I got on my back, lifted my knees, and pulled him onto me. It was easy for him to push and squeeze his boner into me since I was so lubricated, and it was the most delicious sensation I've had down there in ages. He was slipping and sliding around inside me while he was simultaneously ramming against my clit and vulva.

I began feeling like I did when we were first dating, and I kept saying, "I love you Dennis, I love you." And he started saying, "I love you Samantha, I've always loved you," in time to the pumping action of his hips. It was like *pump* "I love you," *pump*, "I love you…"

He reached his hands down the top of my shirt and bra and began squeezing and pulling my nipples just the way I had taught him to. That was something that always makes me start to feel like coming. But I didn't want it all to end yet. I was dying to try out that doggy position we used to enjoy so much now that I was in a super horny mode. I pushed his cock out of me and got onto my knees and leaned over the seats with my naked butt in the air. He slipped in really nicely and came into me right up to the hilt. I could feel his balls slapping against me as he pushed in and out, and my pussy began throbbing and I knew I was going to come really fast.

I hung onto the car seat and pushed myself backwards against Dennis as hard as I could so I could feel rub my pussy against him, and that set him off too. Both of us began climaxing at the exact same time, squirming and pumping against each other. His large squirt of come was shooting into me as both of us grunted and squealed with the ecstasy of it. In the darkness of the van with us linked by our genitals, I felt

Viagra, Sex, & Romance

like we were cocooned in a dark, mysterious lair of sex that nobody else in the world knew about. I was totally satiated.

We both lay around on the floor half naked as we got our breath back. Eventually we sat down on the seats and leaned back to watch the last part of the movie. The Titanic slowly sank away as Dennis held my hand. Celine Dion began singing *My Heart Will Go On* as Dennis looked at me and said, "Samantha - let's remember to do this every once in a while to remind us why we ever got married in the first place." I know he's right.

* * * * *

Tonya

of

Tulsa

VIAGRA PLUS HORMONE SUPPLEMENTS have given our retirement years a new sexual element that I didn't want at first. I didn't even know Viagra would work for women. But, now that I've tried it at the urging of Eddy, my husband, I'm enjoying the effects more than he is. And, bringing good sex back into our lives has given us another benefit we didn't expect - it makes us feel as if we're not really old folks.

My husband and I are in our 70's and we were becoming total couch potatoes. At least when we were younger, we had to run around with our children and grandchildren and our days were pretty active. Since we both retired, we weren't doing much at all for days at a time, and it was starting to make us get really lazy. In fact, the extent of our laziness was becoming ridiculous. At night, and sometimes in the afternoons, we'd read magazines, talk on the phone, and lounge around watching old movies on TV for hours and hours without moving. We hardly even cooked anymore. We'd just order in Chinese food or pizza. We were doing whatever we could to make sure we didn't have to start running around and being busy.

In terms of sex, the energy we put into it had also really decreased. Until we reached our 50's (after 25 years of marriage!) we regularly had intercourse once a week on Sunday, and that suited us fine. Our sexual efforts were never too long or elaborate, but they were enough for our needs and desires. I'd have orgasms without much fuss about half the time, and Eddy was satisfied almost all the time.

When we reached our 60's we slowed down to once a month. Now, in our 70's, Eddy would wake up with a hard-on once in a blue moon, and immediately mount me as quickly as possible. He didn't want to miss any opportunity to get his jollies since he wasn't having that many opportunities, if you know what I mean! But, wouldn't you know it – my Eddy was reading some kind of sexy magazine and decided to try Viagra. And when he found out that it really does make his cock hard whenever he wants, he decided he wanted to get back in the saddle with me every Sunday morning again – or even more if I'd let him! I guess I should have been flattered, but I didn't have much of a desire anymore. And, with both of us rather overweight, and with him bald and me grey, we're not the prettiest sight together, let me tell you. We make sure the blinds are closed and the lights are out so that we aren't able to see too much of each other in our bedroom! I certainly didn't want to increase our lovemaking from our once-a-month routine, Viagra or no Viagra.

I told him, "Eddy, let's not tamper with our happiness. Things are fine the way they are. You don't need to be pulling out your joyrod so often. Life is fine without getting back in the saddle so much! We've done the deed quite enough in our time." If you get my drift, I was trying to get my old stallion to cool his jets.

Eddy, of course, tried every excuse to convince me to let him have his way whenever he wanted. He said, "Tonya, first of all, the more often we have intercourse, the younger and healthier we'll stay. Secondly, I read this important article which says that women experience fewer feminine problems if her husband deposits sperm in her regularly.

"Thirdly, Viagra is the wave of the future. Even Hugh Hefner takes it now, and we're about his age. So we might as well get with it and take it too," he added.

I thought, *what a crock of baloney... who's going to believe all that stuff except for some old coot who's trying to get his rocks off?*

I just didn't feel like accommodating him. I didn't have the same urges I used to when I was younger, so I didn't desire having more sex. It was as simple as that. Then I noticed changes in his habits which made me think twice. Eddy was starting to wear newer clothes. He began hanging around the mall more, and he was spending more time combing the remaining hairs over the top of his head. I suspected he was chasing some other women - and I was right.

One day we drove together to the mall, and he told me to go to the stores I wanted to and he'd meet me later. Instead, I followed him at a distance, and saw him chatting with every saleslady in sight. They all seemed to know him - especially one in particular. She was in the hardware section of Wal-Mart, and they were talking like they were the best of pals. I'd guess she was about 55. She had a nice figure and dyed blonde hair, and they seemed far too familiar for my liking. I thought about confronting them right then and there...

But, as I walked around that store, I looked at myself in the mirror. In that harsh neon light I had to face the truth. I had totally let myself go. Compared to that hussy, I was a mess! I had on stretch black pants which sagged at the knees and rear, a flowery pullover top which looked like a tent cover, and really old-fashioned, big plastic bifocals. To make things worse, I could see my big pot had really grown, and my hair looked like I had slept on it ten times without a shampoo! I thought, *can I blame Eddy for looking around?*

I began trying to figure out how to deal with his new flirting game. I realized that if he used up all his energy at home – if you know what I mean - there'd be nothing left to share with any other woman. As the weeks progressed, I began taking better care of myself. I walked more, shampooed my hair more, put on make-up, and made myself look more like the attractive woman I once was. I began to feel healthier and younger, and I'm sure Eddy began noticing the change.

I also began trying to be more obliging about fulfilling his sexual urges more often, even though it wasn't great for me. Sunday morning would come around, and we'd both go for a walk and then have a shower (in different bathrooms). We'd put on our terry robes and head to the kitchen for coffee and breakfast and the Sunday paper as Eddy took his Viagra. Beore long he'd look at me with a gleam in his eye, then say, "Tonya, I've got something special for you," and lead me by the hand to the bedroom.

He always took off his robe with great pride to reveal his erect manhood sticking straight out from his crotch for all the world to see. I think he was more proud of that thing than he was of having been a vice president at the bank! I must admit it's fun to hold his erection in my hands and feel it as hard and hot as it used to be when we were 25. I get on my back and lie around, trying to be as interested as I can while he does his thing inside me. He's quite good at it, even though we don't try anything fancy. The most strenuous thing we did was to take turns being on top. Within five or ten minutes, he'd have a nice orgasm, although I rarely did. The problem was that my private parts were becoming irritated, and I began to dread our sex sessions.

It was my gynecologist who came to my rescue. He prescribed estrogen supplements along with a special hormonal cream for my vagina, and things suddenly began to get much better. My vagina felt far more receptive and I began to enjoy having his penis inside me, especially now that it was much harder than it had been in years. It meant my clitoris was getting rubbed a lot more, and I had a few good orgasms. I guess it's true what they say about being able to enjoy sex even if you are old! I started to think that maybe Eddy was pretty smart, maybe this new round of lovemaking was good for our health.

Then came the clincher. I started noticing a new trend in all the women's magazines. Many women were finding a great deal of sexual pleasure through Viagra, so I figured, *if my old coot can start to become more horny at 73, why not me?* So, I took one of his pills.

The bottom line is, Viagra turned out to be an excellent aphrodisiac for me too. The sex-enhancing effect was even better than I thought it could be. For me, it meant that my vagina began to feel more receptive and interested in having sex, and that made me want to have intercourse when I took the Viagra. Suddenly, I was doing more than merely keeping up with Eddy - I was wearing him out from time to time! All of a sudden it was me who started suggesting to him that we get it on together, even if it was in the middle of the week. It was much more exciting than lounging around all day doing nothing. At least for that half-hour break we'd feel young and lively. Plus, I began having really nice orgasms almost every time we had intercourse.

After a few months, I decided we needed to spice up our lives and get out of our old routine. Eddy's birthday was approaching, so I figured I'd use that as an excuse to do something special. I had it in my mind to get a new fancy outfit from Victoria's Secret, like all the younger ladies were doing. Partly, I was curious to see if those pretty things could do anything for me despite my shape. And, I wanted to experience something new. I didn't really know what to expect. After all, I am 72! I went to the store, and, as it turns out, the saleslady I dealt with was really nice to me. She suggested an outfit that camouflaged my problem areas in just the right ways. She handed me a baby-blue camisole with lots of lace. Underneath that, I put on a lacy push-up support bra, also in baby-blue, and a pair of baby-blue underpants with Lycra for support. And, for a robe, she handed me a blue silk floor-length kimono. I looked like the Queen of Sheba!

As Eddy's birthday approached, I told him we'd be celebrating it in a special way on Sunday morning. He was curious, but he had no idea what to expect. He asked me if I had a special present for him - and I answered, "I guess you could say that, Eddy!" Little did he know the present was me! We went out for our walk as usual, and we each took one of our pills (I take only half) before heading to the showers. I carefully put on my beautiful new outfit before prancing into the kitchen. I checked myself in a long mirror, and I looked great. I felt sexy and wild again, in a way I hadn't felt for more than 30 years. As for Eddy, when I walked into the kitchen and began singing *Happy Birthday*, that bugger's eyes popped open larger than a pie pan!

His cock shot up straight and hard and poked right out through the front of his bathrobe! He said, "Wow - this is some birthday!" and quickly led me by my hand to the bedroom even before we started having breakfast. He said, "Tonya, we've got to shoot while the ducks are flying!" I thought that was really romantic. I was actually as excited as he was. My new silky outfit felt so sensuous against my skin that it helped make me feel horny. One thing he did - which was amazingly flattering - was to turn the control on the slat blinds so that some light could come into our room. He wanted to watch us screwing!

Eddy asked me for a "Monica Lewinsky" and, since it was his birthday, I obliged. I gave him a nice blow job for a few minutes, and I was really impressed by the stiffness and quality of his erection. It was just as powerful as it had been 25 years ago. I could hardly tell the difference from then, except for the fact that his pubic hair was now grey. Just like the president, he didn't want to come in my mouth, and I was happy about that because I had become very aroused. I knew I'd have a nice, big orgasm pretty quickly if I could get his boner into me.

Eddy pulled off my panties, and told me to leave the rest of my lingerie on while he mounted me because I looked so "cute" in it. I think the last time he called me cute was 30 years ago! I thought it was great fun to keep my long silk robe on, and to feel Eddy fondling my breasts outside my lacy bra.

His cock felt incredible inside me, and he began pumping like he was doing a high-energy aerobics class. I told him I wanted to try a new sex trick I had read about. So, I did this thing of closing my legs while his erection was in me. He, of course, had to spread his legs outside of mine, which was easy to do. We were both pleased and amazed by the new sensation. Because my vagina now felt tighter, it increased the sexual stimulation we both were receiving. It was excellent.

I told him excitedly, "Eddy - don't stop - I'm going to come soon!" He was such a nut - he made me count down to my orgasm, as if I was the space shuttle getting ready for a blast-off. That was a dumb joke he actually started when we were young and they began sending those rockets up to the moon. So I went "10, 9, 8..." and so on until I got to number 4 or 3, and I gave up the count-down as I had the most wicked, pulsating orgasm from deep within my vagina. I was tickled pink about the fact that Eddy was being so playful about sex, just like when we were younger. He, of course, had his own masculine orgasm, grunting like a man possessed... by me.

He said, "Who says we're getting old anyway, Tonya? We don't feel old, do we?" And, I had to agree, I didn't.

So, now we go out more often than we used to. Eddy has gone a bit overboard, prancing around like a young buck at the mall, but that's fine with me. If Hugh Hefner can get away with it, why not Eddy? I mean, let him pretend he's a sexy guy with every store clerk and waitress from here to California - I'm the one who receives his attention. As for me, I also feel more energetic, and I've been losing weight just from being more active and cooking healthier meals instead of ordering all that take-out food with tons of hidden fat. I'll be going back to Victoria's Secret one of these days just so I can keep surprising my old coot. There was no reason for us to accept old age. It's just a number in your head anyway.

* * * * *

Mr. *Virgin*

I LOVE WATCHING MY PENIS GROW when I take Viagra, and that's no joke. My name is Andrew, and I was hardly able to get any kind of hard-on for a whole two years. The sad thing is that my cock worked fine until then, when I was injured in a bad car crash at the age of 25. I ended up with a lot of tissue and nerve damage in the groin. Twenty-five is really young to become impotent. I still had raging sexual urges, but there was no way to put them into action. My sex life consisted of reminiscing about the great times I used to have. A stiff cock and great times always go together, but my cock just couldn't get stiff. I'd just watch everyone from the sidelines and force myself to booze up a lot and pretend I was having as much fun as they were. The good part is that, in the end, being honest about my condition actually helped me find my wife.

Shortly after the accident, I tried praying to make my penis function properly again, but that didn't work (until God helped someone invent Viagra, I guess!) Sometimes I'd think I could look at my penis and use my force of mind to will it to rise, like a snake charmer. I once had a dream after watching an episode of the X-Files that I had developed the power of telekinesis, and that I was able to make my penis start moving just by thinking about it. Of course, no matter how much I stared or willed, it never moved. For these two years, I've stared sadly at my penis as it lay limp between my legs. All it was good for was peeing.

Trying to get a girlfriend was a gigantic problem. I've liked several and they've liked me. I'm tall, I have a good personality, and I have a sense of humor. But they all dropped me pretty quickly after they found out I was damaged that way. Guys have feelings too, and I've cried myself to sleep many nights. I'm not exaggerating when I say I've seriously thought about killing myself. It's not that sex is everything in the world. I have a lot of things I can do for kicks. But without a working cock I can't feel like a real person. Even if you only have sex for 15 minutes once in a million years, it's something that makes you feel alive.

My doctor previously had told me to try old-time aphrodisiacs, like yohimbine or ginseng, but that stuff never did a thing for me. Hell, I would have paid $1,000 for an ounce of rhino horn if I thought it could make me hard! Then, after the FDA approved Viagra, my doctor gave me a prescription for it – and the rest is excellent history.

That first time I took it I began to believe that God really does love us all. Like an age-old memory suddenly emerging into the light of day, my penis, testicles, and scrotum began tingling in a way I had forgotten about years before. I pulled down my pants, lay down on my bed with a pillow propping up my head for a better view, and I just *looked* at my cock. If I had binoculars handy to zoom in on it, I would have used them. There, in front of my eyes, that shrivelled up remnant of my former masculinity was expanding and rising. Once it started, there was no stopping it... it got taller, harder, fatter, until it was as stiff as a baseball bat and pointing straight up into the air like a Patriot missile. I picked up a hand mirror and looked at my very own boner with amazement. From the sides, from the bottom, from the area of my testicles, I checked it out from every angle and it was the most beautiful sight in the world.

I squeezed it in my fist, rubbed it tight between both hands, tickled it and teased it... my old friend was back! If I could have bent over far enough to kiss it, I definitely would have. That first night, I was so self-satisfied that it didn't even occur to me to try and link up with a woman to use it. I just wanted to enjoy the sight. I couldn't resist masturbating myself harder and faster, until I had an orgasm right in my hands. Everything worked - I was a man again.

My first big social event was coming up after I received my prescription, and I told myself, *Andrew, you don't have to fake it anymore, you can do everything that all the other guys do*. It was just my cousin's wedding, but there were going to be some pretty girls there and it was sure to be a fun time.

The following Saturday, while getting ready for the wedding reception, I carefully put a Viagra and a condom in my pocket. Luckily for me, that day I was asked to escort one of the bridesmaids - my cousin's friend, Margaret – who was a real cutie. We had hung out together a few times, but I don't think she had any idea that I really liked her. She's great-looking with long, straight blonde hair, and she loves talking about politics - especially about Clinton and Monica. She was quite a bit shorter than me, at 5'2" - but that's one of the things I found attractive about her. I guess you could say I had a severe inferiority complex during my two years of injury, so I didn't have the confidence to try to get too many dates.

When I picked Margaret up, she was dressed in one of those big puffy dresses they make bridesmaids wear. It was raspberry colored, and it had all sorts of layers and puffy sleeves and shoulders. At least the front was cut pretty low, so you could see the rounded tops of her bosoms in the midst of all that raspberry chiffon. Margaret seemed pretty sheepish in her dress, telling me she thought she looked like a giant birthday cake. I told her she was beautiful – and in fact, she really did look beautiful with nice make-up around her eyes, pink lipstick, pretty earrings, and her hair flowing down to her shoulders. She smelled wonderful with some really sexy kind of perfume. If I hadn't been damaged in that stupid accident, I would have been hard all night starting from the moment she got into my car!

The wedding ceremony and dinner went fine. Margaret sat beside me at dinner, and we were joking and talking a lot about politics, our jobs, and other stuff. The band started playing, and Margaret asked me to dance, and that too was lots of fun. We did some fast ones, and a couple of slow ones where we hung on to each other. From my viewpoint, which was about ten inches above hers, I could practically look right down her dress at her amazing breasts. I tried not to be too obvious, but I'm sure she knew I admired her in all ways.

I decided to pop a Viagra right then. I wanted to feel like a normal man and I wanted her to think I was normal! And, in case we'd end up making out later, there was absolutely no way I wanted to find myself in the horrible position of not having a hard-on. Even if she had no desire to be sexual with me, I didn't want it to be me who had to back out and be embarrassed. I had enough of that! I figured if

worst came to worst, I could masturbate later on if I had to
make my penis go down.

As they were serving coffee and wedding cake, my
boner made a reappearance. I even had to reach into my
pocket as I used to do in the old days and discreetly shift it
over to the side so it would feel more comfortable. The music
started up again, and when we danced to the next slow
number, my boner began pressing against her hip bone.
Margaret turned her eyes up to me quizzically, but I wasn't
surprised about what she said next. I knew everyone was
talking about me since my accident. She said, "Andrew - I
guess you don't really have that problem everyone says you
do. In fact, you sure don't feel like you have any problem at
all!"

Privately, my heart was humming, but all I said in reply
was simply, "Nope, I don't."

Margaret and I were pressed up totally close to each
other and my hard-on was undeniably rubbing against her, just
as much as her breasts were rubbing against me. I had the
feeling from the little moves she made while we danced that
she was deliberately trying to hold herself closer to me. It was
wonderful. That was when I began falling in love with her. I
should have felt great since it was all so nice and she was right
there close to me, but I was nervous. I knew it was only the
Viagra which was allowing me to develop my erection. I felt I
had to be honest and tell her so, because I wanted her to trust
me totally. I didn't want her to find out later that I lied about
still being crippled that way. I knew my confession might have
caused her to dump me, but I decided to lay it on the line. If
we were going to develop a relationship, we'd have to make
sure we didn't lie to one another.

When the song ended, I took her off to the side of the hall and said, "Margaret – you may not know this, but I have feelings for you. I always have, but now I feel even stronger about it. But I do still have a problem. It's only my medication that's making me normal again. In fact, I took one of my pills tonight just so I can feel normal like all the other guys."

Right away, she guessed I was taking Viagra. She took my hand and squeezed it, then looked in my eyes and said, "That's sweet of you to tell me, Andrew, but you'd be totally special to me with or without Viagra, and nothing else matters. I know I have feelings for you too."

Woah! My heart just melted. We stayed close to each other and held hands for the rest of the night. I'm sure my cousin (the bride) noticed us together, and when she threw the bouquet she aimed it to Margaret, who caught it and then turned beet red.

I drove her back to her parents' house where she was living. I parked the car at the door and we began kissing. Those were the most delicious kisses I've ever experienced. She took my hand and put it on her breast, and she felt totally warm and luscious. The funny thing was, I didn't want to go too far. Margaret was more forward than I was, and she moved her hand around my crotch, caressing my hard-on. Although it felt wonderful, I suddenly found myself saying, "You know, Margaret, we don't have to rush anything. I like you too much to mess anything up with us by going too far too fast."

She started laughing in a relieved kind of way. "That's so nice - I was worried you wouldn't like me unless we had sex because you'd get really frustrated in your present condition."

It was great that we were talking openly, and I told her that since I already liked her, she didn't have to worry about my condition. She added, "Now that we've got that out of the way, come in for a Coke."

I had an enormous feeling of relief from the fact that there wasn't any pressure on us anymore. We had our Cokes sitting around the kitchen table, laughing and talking, and it felt totally natural to be with her. We went downstairs to the basement to watch the late news on TV. By then everyone else in the house was asleep, and we sat around on some cushions on the carpet. I think we could have kept on talking until the sun came up!

I still had my boner, but I was trying to ignore it. I think Margaret was able to see it every time I stood up or moved around, and she actually asked me if she could touch it. I said sure, and she began caressing it again on top of my pants, as if she was very curious about it. I told her no woman had touched me there for two years, and she laughed and said, "So, Andrew, that means you're a born-again virgin!" I laughed too. At that point, I think she was starting to see me as some sort of challenge.

She began to really tease me. "Mr. Virgin, do you want to see my fancy underwear? You can look, but only if you don't touch…"

Margaret stood up, then lifted her big flouncy raspberry dress right up to her waist and then up and over her head. Underneath, she had on a pink lace bra, the sexiest pink garter thing I've ever seen to hold up her nylons, and underneath that a pair of pink lace panties. She was definitely succeeding in making me go nuts. She kneeled down right in front of me and my body temperature must have risen by 200 degrees! She was the most beautiful sight I have ever seen – like an angel who was just un-gift-wrapped for me. I began kissing her bosom all over, sliding my hands down into the top of her bra, and stroking her nipples with my fingertips. They became erect and pointy, and I slid my hands around her and undid her bra, so that her breasts were totally free in my hands. Seeing her naked and smelling her perfume was making me wild. I licked and kissed her breasts, then her shoulders, and then her body all the way down to just above her pubic hair.

Margaret undid all the buttons on my shirt, and, when I was bare, she gently lowered her breasts to touch my chest. She undid my zipper and belt, and helped me pull off my pants. Then I undid the snaps of her garters, and took off her underwear. Even her pussy smelled delicious, as if she had put a drop of perfume in there just to be sure.

I was so involved in looking at her, I didn't even notice my boner. But there it was! Big and strong, and pointing up like the Statue of Liberty. She started sucking my cock like a lollipop, and I felt like I was being reborn. I felt so lucky, having love and sex at the same time. I caressed Margaret's vagina, and swirled her clit with my fingers. She was the most womanly woman I had ever been with, and I felt as if we belonged together forever. My cock seemed to be growing hotter in her mouth with every beat my heart. She stroked my erection several times with her hands, and then I couldn't stop myself at all – my cock gushed out glorious pulses of come into her pink-lipsticked mouth. I had such an overwhelming feeling of release, it was as if a two-year nightmare of frustration had suddenly come to an end. Maybe that fantastic sexual experience helped me fall in love with her, but I don't think so. I was in love with her anyway.

I admit my eyes got misty. "I haven't been like this with a girl for so long. I feel so good, it's like I have to thank you." She put her finger on my lips, and said, "Andrew, ssssh – you already did. I enjoyed it as much as you did."

My boner wasn't about to go down yet. And, Margaret still seemed eager to continue, which I thought was an excellent idea. So, I took out the condom I brought with me, put it on, turned over onto my back, and asked Margaret to lie on top of me. I wanted her to be in control of everything, so that she could be as satisfied as possible. She looked me right in the eye as she straddled me and began kissing me with deep tongue kisses. She said, "I know this is important for you, Mr. Virgin - and it's important for me to. I really want to be your first girl." Then, holding my boner at the entrance to her vagina, she pointing it in and settled down on top of it. I thought, *yes, this is wonderful, this must be love.*

Our screwing felt amazing, better than I had imagined it could during my two-year absence from this field of dreams. I never wanted our intercourse to end, and, in fact, I felt as if I could screw her forever. She was moving her hips in a steady rhythm, making my cock move in and out of her, squeezing it tight with her vagina with every movement. I was able to last a long time since I had already come, and I tried to match her rhythm of movement until she started coming herself. She clutched me really tightly, then practically began screaming from the intensity. I was freaked that her parents might wake up, so I put my hand up to close her mouth and she tried to stifle herself as much as possible. It was pretty obvious she enjoyed it as much as I did!

Even after she climaxed, my cock was still inside her, so I helped her turn over onto her back and began screwing her in the good old missionary position. It was wonderful for me because I was able to look into her eyes and squeeze and lick her breasts while I was fucking away. I too came again, and while I was moaning and emoting, we heard footsteps on the stairs, and we could tell a light went on in the kitchen above us. We realized it must have been one of her parents.

I pulled out of her quickly, and we both grabbed our clothes fast. She threw her dress on without any underwear, and I ran into the bathroom with all my stuff. It was her dad all right, and he walked right down to the basement. I dressed really quickly, splashed water on my face, and came out pretending nothing had happened. I think he fell for it, but I never was sure he did.

We made small talk with him for a few minutes by talking about the wedding reception we had just been to. Then, he told Margaret it was time to walk me to my car, and he went back up to bed. Margaret and I let out a huge sigh of relief, and started hugging and laughing.

"Well," she said, "for a virgin you did really well."

I answered, "So – you've got my cherry – that means you have to marry me now!"

"I think I will," she said with a smile.

I said, "You're not scaring me, you know."

She said, "You're not supposed to get *scared.* "

When we said goodnight at my car, we kissed each other only lightly in case her dad was snooping on us. We did hug each other really tight.

Three months later, together with our parents, we hosted our official engagement party.

We both knew that her girlfriends thought there was something wrong with me, and they could never figure out why she always looked so happy with me. I would have told them "Viagra" - but it was more than that. It was love.

* * * * *

Chuck and Larry

in

Nevada

MY PAL LARRY AND I have known each other since we were in the navy during the 50's. We had great wild times back then whenever we were on leave in foreign ports. The Yankee dollar, then as now, could buy you anything in the world. Especially important to us was the fact that we were able to buy the services of some of the most beautiful girls in the world wherever we went. The attractions were booze and sex, and the more you could get, the higher you scored.

When our tours of duty were over, we found wives and settled down in different states, he in Louisiana and me in Wisconsin. But we've managed to stay in touch and to meet during the odd business trip. We'd always talk about our fondest memories, of the great whores and the amazing adventures we shared together. We'd say, "hey, we've got to do it all again someday." But that was just a crazy dream. We had children to raise and wives to keep happy. Until now, that is. Both of us have been divorced for several years, the kids have families of their own, and now we've got free time *and* available money. We began dreaming up the idea of meeting in Vegas and making a tour of the legal whorehouses to sample the delights there. Well, my motto in life is, "You regret more the things you don't do than the things you do." So, I convinced Larry that the time was *now.* And off we went for one of the greatest weekends we've ever had in our lives!

We spent the first night hanging around the casinos, but neither of us was into gambling. There were many "working girls" lurking around, but the hotels were too harsh and business-like for us, so we decided to go to the finer whorehouses to look for the kind of women we were after.

I've always been pretty good at sex, even as I got older. I didn't ask Larry what kind of shape he was in. But I told him I was bringing along my bottle of Viagra. I had taken it a few times already with a girlfriend I had, and it really worked wonders for me. For the kind of weekend we were planning to have, Viagra was going to be the drug of choice. We rented a car in the morning and drove past the glittering casinos of Vegas to some of the finest brothels in the world. And, where some of the finest women in the world were ours for the choosing.

Our first stop, the Roaming Rabbit Ranch, had about 30 women - and almost all were beauties! Our eyes popped open when we hung around the bar. There were gorgeous women of every description wherever we turned. "Hey Chuck," Larry said, "aren't you beginning to feel like a kid in a candy store?" We looked at each other with big smiles. We wanted all of them. We sat down for a drink to take in the sights in the spacious lobby. There was a pool table and some couches where customers and women were sitting around, smoking, drinking and talking.

Right away, I spotted the woman I wanted to choose first. She was a vivacious, smiley blond who was the opposite of my ex-wife, who had become rather overweight and mean-looking before our break-up. This honey was full-breasted with a thin waist and long legs. She was wearing a tight white leotard top - without a bra! – and white short-shorts. I couldn't help admiring her large breasts, and the way her nipples clearly showed right through her top. But more than that, I couldn't stop staring at the way her full red lips moved as she spoke, the way her green eyes gleamed when she smiled, and the way she flung her long, wavy hair around to get it away from her face. Larry looked at me and laughed. "I think you've found true love," he said. I told him he was right.

It was like a dream come true. I was going to be able to take her naked in my arms and feel her breasts and cunt pressing against me. She might even suck my cock. She'd do anything I wanted, guaranteed, as long as I paid her, of course. But parting with a few bucks wasn't much of a penalty to have my dreams fulfilled! Larry picked a long-legged black-haired beauty who looked a lot like Cher. I said, "Larry - I'm worried you might end up marrying this one!"

We were both a little nervous because we hadn't done this kind of whoring around for 30 years, but neither of us were going to need any Viagra for our first fuck. If we didn't get hard-ons with these babes, we might as well forget about living! We began politely circling our chosen women to show we were interested and soon began talking to them. Mine told me her name was Suzanne, while Larry's was Jade. For about ten minutes they talked to us in a way that made us feel we were the most important people in the world to them. Then we paid out our $250 each for an hour of their time, and we went to separate rooms upstairs.

Suzanne peeled off her tight white top when we were alone, and she was suddenly naked in front of me – and she was beautiful. I loved looking at her bountiful, uplifted bosom with her firm nipples staring at me. She came over to me and stood inches away. "You can touch me, Chuck, you know. I like you," she said. I smiled, and reached out to caress her breasts, and they felt warm and womanly and sweet as a creampuff in my hands. I could have just played with them for an hour and I would have been happy. Then, she peeled off her short shorts and her red g-string, and she noticed that I was nervously staring at the closely-shaved patch of bush she had covering her cunt. She took my hand and pressed it onto her, and I let a finger slip inside her to feel her warmth and wetness as I caressed her. I was quite taken with her, and being able to touch her like that felt as good as any experience I had in my Navy days.

Suzanne undid my zipper, and pulled out my cock. I was hard and eager for her. I leaned back on the couch as she put a condom on me. Then, she straddled me, and aimed my boner into her cunt. That was when I became really overwhelmed – she felt so hot and wet and tight, and her breasts were bopping around in front of my face... and I climaxed in two minutes flat! It was nice coming into her, but that meant our session was over, and that made me sad. Just before I pulled my cock out, she started faking some noises as if she was climaxing. But I told her not to bother, that I was happy with everything just the way it was. She kissed me quickly on the cheek, and before I knew it I was back down in the bar – where Larry soon followed. "It was great, but really fast," I told him. And he admitted it was true for him too. Neither of us wanted to rush away because we loved the feeling of sex that was in the club, so we went to their small restaurant and had a couple of sandwiches.

"Larry – now's the time for our Viagra," I said. He had never tried it until then, but he took one when I did, and by the time we finished our lunch, we were both raring to go again.

Suzanne was in a corner of the bar, and my heart was beating fast. I didn't care about all the other women there, I wanted her again, so I sauntered over and told her so. She said with genuine surprise, "That's so nice, Chuck, but are you sure you're ready for me again?" I told her she'd find out soon for herself!

We entered a nice room with a view of the desert, and she was about to find out that I was more ready than she had imagined. I took off my pants and I had one of the nicest, hardest boners I've ever had in my life. She looked at it and smiled wide, "I guess your nick-name should be 'Mr. Stud.' That's quite a pistol you've got there!"

I liked her playfulness, but I wanted to fuck her good and hard, and with the help of my Viagra boner, I did that it in spades. I put on a condom and she lay down naked on her back on the bed with her shapely legs spread out for me. At the center of the big Y shape formed by her legs was her beautiful pussy. I could see it perfectly from that angle, with its little pink lips and her pearl of a pink clit poised on top. The light veil of pubic hair framed her vagina perfectly, and I touched her gently before entering her. I think she liked my touch because she sighed deeply a few times as I caressed her vagina with one hand, and squeezed each breast in turn with the other.

My boner was seeking action, and my heart was pounding. I was really turned on. I thought, "Man, I'm lucky, I'm going to start fucking one of the most beautiful women I've ever seen! If I was younger, I would have married her." I got on top of her and the tip of my cock quickly found its way into her beautiful pussy. I began fucking her with long, slow strokes, trying to make it last as long as possible. Suzanne looked at me with a knowing smile, "I know you must be on Viagra, but it sure feels nice to me."

I asked her if she'd turn around so I could screw her doggy-style, and she said, "Sure – you've paid for an hour, you can screw me from any angle you want, Chuck!" I was glad she remembered my name. She did turn over, and I was able to hold her heart-shaped ass in my hands and look at the slimness of her waist as I slipped my cock in from behind her. I continued making my long, slow strokes in and out. I wanted it to go on forever. She began shaking her ass, and the sensations of her pussy rubbing against my cock made me hotter and more excited by the minute.

I asked her to do one more position, this time back on my lap on the couch, so I could see her breasts at eye level, and she graciously obliged. Suzanne kneeled around my waist as I sat there, and she played with my penis a little, squeezing it from the base to the tip. Then she eased her pussy down on me and made cute circular movements on my cock. She started whispering in a sexy deep voice, "Chuck, don't you feel like coming, don't you want your cock to shoot off your hot come right into my pussy, don't you, Chuck?"

All I could do was nod my head in agreement. She reached between my legs from behind her, and began tickling my balls and scratching them lightly with her nails. She was swinging her hips fast, left and right, and brushing her breasts around on my face. That was it for me, and my sperm went zooming out of cock as I climaxed into her cunt. She could see I was flushed with satisfaction, and she slowly rose off me and handed me the box of Kleenex to wrap up the used condom. She said, "Chuck, it's swell doing business with you," and I think she meant it. I know I paid her a total of $500 for less than two hours of her time, but it's possible she found me a bit nicer than the other guys who come by.

Larry was already down at the bar, and he had the biggest grin I'd ever seen. "I picked that red-head over there – she looks just like my wife did when we got engaged. She gave me a great blow job at first, and then I screwed her good – and instead of complaining about money, or whatever, like my wife used to do, she thanked me," he said, laughing.

We drove off into the sunset feeling like the triumphant, footloose team of Butch Cassidy and the Sundance Kid, happy with our experience and ready for more action later on during the weekend. We went to relax at our motel for awhile, and we ended up conking out completely for the night. We weren't used to so much action in a long time! After sleeping in late, we grabbed some lunch and another Viagra, then went to a resort-style whorehouse in the area called Madame Bell's. There were many lovely-looking women there, but none struck me the way Suzanne did. She just had that special something that really attracted me.

I was drawn to a couple of Oriental woman who looked just like these beautiful Thai girls I had screwed on a memorable night in Bangkok 40 years ago. Both were nubile and young looking, one on the slim side and the other a bit chubby. Neither seemed older than 21. I had a great idea for screwing them both simultaneously, and they happily agreed. My cock was already feeling great, so I knew I was up for it.

As the three of us walked down the hall, it seemed like another dream was coming true.

When they took off their clothes, they were even more attractive than I had imagined. They had beautiful olive colored skin, which seemed almost too beautiful to touch – but I touched them all right! They were very amenable to my suggestions (at $250 each for the hour, why wouldn't they be!) and I first requested that we do nice massages.

They lay down beside each other on the bed, and I stroked my hands all over their breasts, butts, and pussies. Then, they both got up and massaged me at the same time. I was really excited as I admired their pretty faces and figures, and thought how pampered I felt right then. The slim one was more giggly, and she lingered over my balls and boner as she massaged me, joking to the chubbier one about how hard and hot I was for such an old geezer. To me, this was like the adult version of DisneyWorld. Here I was, this 66-year-old son-of-a-gun with two beautiful women ready to oblige my every whim and please me any way I wanted. I was really excited because I knew I would be acting out one of my favorite sexual daydreams.

After that touchy-feely stuff, I was ready for the real thing. I had both of them lie side by side on the bed with their knees up towards their chest, so that their lovely little vaginas were totally accessible to me and my cock. Their pussies smelled like musk, and it made me feel like I wanted to start screwing right away. The woman on my left was the slimmer one, and she was the one I wanted to do first. I got on my knees facing both sets of hips and cunts, put on a condom, and then began fucking the slim one nice and slowly while I took turns caressing all four breasts. After a couple of minutes screwing her, I pulled out my cock and pushed it into the chubbier woman's vagina for another couple of minutes and did the slow fuck with her. Meanwhile, I continued caressing all four of their breasts. It was quite a pleasure for me to take a few turns screwing one, then the other, while my cock got hotter and hotter.

I knew I could have exploded in a climax at any moment, but there was one more part of my fantasy to fulfil. I asked the women to turn over and get on their hands and elbows and lift up their rear ends. It was a pleasure to see the sight of these two beautiful butts - one big and rounded, the other slim and muscular. And both were there for my viewing, screwing, and touching pleasure. Both women's cunts were now easily accessible to me from behind, and that was where I was aiming to please myself. Still on my knees behind them, I felt like a wild, powerful dog as I fucked the chubby one hard from behind, and then screwed the slim one, moving as slow or fast as I pleased with each of them. They obligingly responded with their own hip movements, swaying in time to me. It was much more exciting than any kind of roller coaster ride or any other wild adventure I could ever think of!

When I couldn't hold back for even one more second, I came inside the slim one with a super-powerful gush that made her laugh some more. I dropped down onto the bed, quite spent from that superlative sexual experience. The girls got up and turned on the shower and invited me to join them since there was about 15 minutes left for the hour. I just jumped right in and we all soaped each other and rinsed off together, and it was great fun. But there was no more hanky panky for me that day – my cock needed a rest! I thanked the women and they suggested I give each of them an extra tip for their obliging service, so I gave each of them an additional

$50, for which they nicely thanked me. I went back down to meet Larry.

He was already waiting, smiling and sipping a beer. He said he had a wonderful fuck with another large redhead who gave him a fine story about how she was a nice girl from New England who had fallen on hard times. We were both pretty satiated, and spent the rest of the day playing the slots and hanging around at our motel pool.

I had one more goal in mind before returning home. I wanted to see Suzanne again, not so much to fuck her, but to talk with her and be alone with her. What can I say – I liked her. So the next day before leaving we drove back to the first whorehouse. I was a bit sad because she was nowhere to be found. Larry and I already had boners from taking another (our last) Viagra, so we did quickies – me with a Baywatch beauty look-alike, and he with another redhead. We had reached our limit and were ready to return home!

Larry and I sadly said good-bye at the airport to each other before boarding different planes, promising we'd get together again soon. We were two old guys who were happy to have been able to pretend we were young again. And, if memory serves me well, it was as good now as it was then. Who says you can't turn back the hands of time? I know for sure that you can at least bend them back for a little while!

* * * * *

my

Church Beauty

WE WOULD HAVE BECOME a happily married couple with or without Viagra. My wife, Megan, and I found our own nice ways to cope with my problem. But, being able to take Viagra when we feel like it gives me confidence that Megan will never feel she's missing anything by not having sex the way everyone else does. Our story shows that making ourselves happy without Viagra might have been a blessing in disguise for us.

My name is Taylor and I'm only 31. I've suffered with impotency ever since I was a teenager. My problem is that my hard-ons are almost always too soft to be of much use. It's tough to live with this condition. I was always scared that people would make fun of me if they knew, and I was always worried that I would never be able to find love with a woman. My first wife, Charlene, left me because of my problem - something that shook me to my roots. Last year, when I met my new fiancee, Megan, I was so nervous about explaining my impotency to her that I practically threw up.

Psychiatrists and physicians were always telling me that the problem was all in my head – if I'd only relax more, or concentrate more, or drink more caffeine, I'd be able to produce an erection. But I knew the problem wasn't in my head, because my head was certain that I wanted sex. I knew I wanted to have sexual intercourse with women, but erections just didn't happen.

Five years ago, I rushed into marriage with Charlene. Many "experts" said everything would work out in the sex department after we married as long as we had love for each other. But they were wrong. I was devastated when Charlene told me she was leaving me after two years. She said the fact that I was impotent obviously meant I didn't find her attractive, so there was no reason for us to stay together. I tried to tell her the problem wasn't my soul, which truly loved her. My problem was my body, which didn't respond physically to my feelings. But my words fell on deaf ears.

Despite my impotency, I always tried to do the right thing for her by making her have orgasms through cunnilingus and manual penetration. But she said she still wasn't satisfied. I developed a lot of anxiety since all of my romantic efforts were never good enough for her. The way Charlene put it, there was no point to even cuddling or making out because the sex would end up being lousy. And it certainly wasn't getting any better as time went by. I became petrified about trying any type of sexual activity with her since I'd probably end up limp and she'd end up exasperated. I didn't mind not having orgasms myself, as long as I had her love. Then I lost that.

During those two years of marriage, our arguments grew more frequent, and when she finally announced she was divorcing me, she said there was just no point in even discussing it anymore.

Since Viagra hadn't yet been invented, I couldn't try it. There were these injections you could give yourself in the penis, or a dumb-looking vacuum tube you could shove on top of your cock to make an erection, but those things seemed so artificial and unGodly.

Finally, I met Megan, my current fiancee, in 1996 in our church. She and I grew close through our volunteer work with handicapped children. She was a really pretty redhead with lots of freckles, and she had this cute way of scrunching up her little button nose when she laughed, which she did often. Plus, she's a wonderful person.

I was deeply impressed by the way she encouraged the crippled kids to cope with their wheelchairs and other devices. Our work involved taking out one handicapped child together each weekend for an afternoon trip. Being together so often made us really appreciate each other. For me, it was delightful being with such a bright, optimistic, caring woman – who also was lots of fun. The kids absolutely adored Megan, and soon, so did I. She was everything I wanted and hoped for in a woman. I knew she wanted children of her own, and I couldn't think of a better mother for my future children. So, I asked her to accept me as her husband, and I gave her a ring on my bended knee that Christmas. I was relieved and thrilled that she lovingly accepted my proposal.

Megan shared my religious beliefs about not having sex before marriage, so she didn't yet know about my impotence. I dreaded having to tell her, but I knew I would eventually have to so that we could find out if we could deal with it as a couple. If Viagra had existed, I wouldn't have had to make such a big deal about my impotency, but who knew a drug like that was going to be invented? I certainly didn't want to go through all the pain of getting divorced ever again. And, I didn't want to mislead Megan. One good point I verified with my doctor was that I would be able to father a child through a process of collecting my sperm and fertilizing her eggs at the right time in her cycle. So at least that part of our marriage would be okay.

The fateful day arrived when we had to set the date of our wedding, and I finally started telling her about my impotence. I said, "Megan, I've been too scared to mention this before, but I know I have to say this now before you make your final commitment to marry me. I'll always find a way to keep you satisfied sexually and spiritually, but we may have to be intimate in a different way because intercourse doesn't always work for me." Then, I added I'd totally accept her decision if she wanted to break things off at that very moment. My life, my love, my everything hung in limbo. Her response was almost immediate.

Megan put her arms around my neck, kissed me on the mouth, and said, "I love you, Taylor, and you love me – we can trust in God to help us find a way to be happy together."

I almost began bawling from relief and joy. Then, I added, "I know God helps those who help themselves, so we'll find the ways we can to make each other happy." I was *determined* to avoid the situation I had been in with Charlene, when my problem grew into a giant fiasco.

During the time which we have since named as "BV" – Before Viagra – Megan and I learned what we could about sexual dysfunction with the old-fashioned self-help sex manuals of that earlier era. They were pretty basic, but they did offer advice on how to achieve orgasm without penetration. Since we weren't going to have sexual penetration anyway before our wedding, we thought we should begin experimenting so that we could perfect our techniques in advance. At that time we still partly believed the stuff the doctors were saying about relaxing and getting in the mood. So, at first we did the recommended things like simply taking off our clothes and lying around naked with each other.

I know I would have had a total orgasm if I was normal just from watching her undress that first time because she was so beautiful. It was a sunny Sunday afternoon after church, and we were cuddling and kissing tenderly on my living room carpet. "I guess now's the time," Megan said as she stood up with the sweetest, most innocent expression on her cute face I've ever seen. She scrunched up her nose in that way of hers, then, with a look of determination, undid the buttons on her baby blue sweater to reveal her white sports bra underneath. She took everything off above the waist and stood there with her large, firm breasts inches away from me. She said, "Now, Taylor, you take off your shirt." I didn't need any urging. I took it off immediately and we lay down together, and it was beautiful. That was our first venture of sexual touching with each other, simply lying with her breasts touching my chest as we talked and kissed.

In the coming days, we graduated to taking off all our clothes and touching each other everywhere. It was quite a delight to see, touch, and smell her lightly perfumed vagina. We began massaging each other, but we didn't even try to have orgasms. She'd massage me, rub my penis and testicles, and then rub my back and legs and so on. If I did actually get a hard-on, she'd squeeze it and caress it, then tickle my balls, and then just lie back and relax. Our goal was to avoid making a big deal of an erection one way or another. When it was my turn, I'd massage Megan's breasts and the rest of her lovely body. She'd smile as my hands wandered over her luscious skin or tickled her belly-button. I liked to linger on her soft delta-shaped mound of pubic hair, and stroke her thighs all the way down to her feet. We also took showers and a bubble bath together so that we could become familiar with each other in non-sexually-threatening ways.

As the next week progressed, we graduated to using oral stimulation to arouse each other, and then we began to see what type of orgasm (if any) we could produce for the other. When it was her turn, she'd lick my cock and rub it vigorously with various creams to try to keep my erection stiff for as long as possible.

I started by kissing her deeply on the mouth, and then moving my lips and tongue down along her neck. I'd lick each breast and nipple in turn, then lick her tummy and belly button, and then move my tongue onto her quivering pearl-shaped clit at the top of her vagina. I loved caressing her sensuous butt and the small of her back while I was doing cunnilingus on her, and she really liked it too. After this exercise, I began inserting one or two fingers into her pussy.

The following Sunday, I went quite a lot further. I put my mouth onto her entire pussy, manipulating both sides of her vulva and her clit in my mouth in a rhythmical sucking action. Her pussy tasted so nice to me, like it had a hint of vanilla. Megan began moving her vagina up and down against my mouth in the same rhythm, and soon she started coming like she had seen the glory. When she came, her vagina released cute extra little spurts of flowery-tasting stuff.

I was relieved and excited to make her come so well, and I was really turned on by it myself. I had developed a pretty nice erection. Megan started trying to make me come right after she did by sucking on my cock, but I stopped her. I didn't want her to think she was obligated to make me have an orgasm just because she had one. It really wasn't that important to me, and I wanted her to know that. I just loved doing all this with her. I loved her and cherished her and all I could do was pray that she was as happy as I was.

A few days later I stopped in at a sex boutique to look for sex toys. I decided to buy a small dildo with long bunny-shaped ears at the base which could be used to tie it onto someone's waist. I guessed it was really made for lesbians to use with each other, but I thought this would be one alternate means for us to have sex too. I also bought a pair of fluffy, furry, mittens which I thought might feel good as part of some manual stimulation for either of us.

The results were better than I could have predicted. Megan didn't want me to penetrate her with the bunny dildo because it might interfere with her hymen even if it wasn't technically sexual intercourse. But I got it buzzing, and just from rubbing it around on the outside of her vagina and clitoris she quickly reached a really nice orgasm. I liked the way she looked at me right in the eyes as she came, as if she wanted me to know how intense she felt. She was panting, and her breasts were rising up and down as she smiled at me. "Taylor - I don't think we'll have to worry too much about sex after we're married, dear," she said. That, of course, was music to my ears.

In turn, Megan put the furry mitts on her hands which made her look like she had abominable snowman paws. We laughed as she rubbed the fur up and down on my penis. She licked the tip of my cock whenever it emerged from the fur. I was erect all right, and I'm sure I was stiffer than I've ever been in my life. I suddenly experienced the first orgasm I had through her intervention, and it was tremendous. It was like that old Hemingway line about the earth moving because I felt like I was in the middle of an earthquake as my come shot out of me. We had discovered there definitely are many ways to satisfy one another sexually without intercourse, and that made us confident about the future together. It also erased many of my fears about getting close to a woman.

We experimented with several other sex toys after that. One really good one was a vibrating cock ring which went around the base of my penis and helped to maintain it hard while Megan sucked my tip and caressed my shaft. For fun, I also bought a pair of handcuffs, and we take turns using them on each other while we pleasure the other.

So, we married in the spring, and we were jubilant with love on our wedding night. That night, we used our toys and our experience to have a beautiful experience of penetration and orgasm. Megan placed the vibrating cock ring down to the base of my penis, then stroked my cock and licked it, and I achieved an erection that was as stiff as wood!

I entered her vagina for the first time, and the vibrating cock ring helped keep me stiff and aroused until I came inside her with a wonderful shooting climax. Megan could feel my ejaculation inside her vagina, and she began hugging me and kissing me because we were both so happy about it. The vibrations of the cock ring against her clitoris soon set off her own orgasm. It was a truly spiritual evening, and a great start to a really happy marriage.

In the following months, sometimes I could manage penetration, and sometimes not. I'd find ways to make her climax, and she'd do things to make come one way or another. Whatever we did, we were happy because we loved being together. Using sex toys or manual and oral stimulation to bring each other to a climax is just as good as any kind of penetration. All of it was fun, and it's been a great marriage.

Viagra, as everyone knows, burst onto the scene in the spring of 1998, which was after Megan and I had been married for more than a year. I made an appointment with a urologist to see if he thought Viagra would be good for me. He actually told me I may as well skip the expensive test to determine if I was experiencing poor blood flow in my groin. Instead, he simply wrote me a prescription for Viagra and told me I might as well try it now that such a drug was available. If it didn't work, then he'd do the diagnostic procedure later and we'd evaluate those results.

Well, as I guess a zillion other men have found out, I did achieve much better erections right away. On the first night we tried it, I believe I made Megan pregnant! I sure came a lot, deep inside her, and that must have done the trick. I just took one of the pills before we went to bed, and as we lay around talking and watching TV, my erection sprang up all on its own. It was stiff enough to actually hold the sheet in the air, and, when I noticed it, I nudged Megan and we both gasped. My cock was actually pointing straight up in the air.

Megan said, "Taylor, we shouldn't let it go to waste."

I was happy that my erection was so strong and viable for once that Megan would be able to just use it any way she wanted without worrying that it would start to droop. For a few minutes, she turned around and we did 69 together, and then she grabbed my erection in her hands, mounted me and inserted it straight into her vagina as she rode me like a rocking horse. My cock felt wonderful inside her, but more importantly, my soul felt excellent to see her enjoying our marriage the way a woman is supposed to.

She had an orgasm before I did, and she had a big smile on her face as she was groaning and panting on top of me. We laughed, and cuddled, and she asked me if I wanted her to bring me to orgasm with her mouth or the fur mitts before my hard-on went away. But I really didn't want that - I wanted her to get back on top of me again and use me some more and take advantage of this opportunity.

She did climb back on top of me again, and this time her rocking action and the deep penetration of my cock inside her made me come in a fascinating, sparkling ejaculation. She became so juicy down there from all my come and hers, that she was able to slide her pussy around in circles on me with my cock still inside her. Her hips were making circle patterns in one direction, and then the other, and then she started doing little circle 8's on me. It was so much fun to watch her breasts bouncing away as she wriggled and writhed on me. She soon had another orgasm just before my erection subsided, and we lay in each other's arms smiling and hugging.

Megan is quite pregnant now, and we're happy about that. But I want to point out that we only use Viagra once a month or so, simply because we totally enjoy all the other ways we've found of stimulating each other without intercourse. We're really glad we had the opportunity - or the need - to experiment before falling into a routine of just doing penetration. Using some of our sex toys and other means of stimulation has meant that we get to enjoy each other's bodies in many different ways. And that's what I recommend for all married couples as a way of avoiding getting into a rut in your sexual routine. Just because you can have sexual penetration, it's not the only thing you should do. I guarantee that your wife or husband will enjoy any new experiments you try.

* * * * *

the *Paris*

of

North America

THE REAL PARIS would have been too expensive for my husband and I to afford for our Christmas vacation, so we took the next best choice - Montreal, Canada. This city is nicknamed the Paris of North America because everything's French there - the signs, the way people talk, even the way they dress and act. It's really charming and different. My goal was to change our environment as much as possible so we could really feel as if we were starting our life anew.

God knows we needed a change.

My name is Eleanor. My hsuband, Lewis, and I are nearing 50. We've been beside ourselves with grief for the past year because our oldest son, Ricky, was killed in a car crash. Ricky was in his final semester at college when he got into a car with a drunken friend after a New Year's party. The friend

Viagra, Sex, & Romance

drove into a tree at 60 mph. He walked away without a scratch, but Ricky died right there. We never had the chance to say goodbye to him, or to tell him how much we loved him.

Our family suffered as we buried him and during the months that followed. But as I watched my other three children cope with the pain, I realized that Lewis and I had to pull ourselves together. We had to resume our roles as the parents that those three kids needed to keep their lives on track. We had to become a couple again.

Lewis just wasn't able to put the pain behind him. He became sullen and solitary and rarely talked at all to me. He never made love with me, not a single time, for the whole 12 months. I don't think he achieved a single erection in all that time. He and I were in big trouble, and I insisted we go to a couples' psychologist. The psychologist's message was that we had to change our mindset, especially during Christmas, because that was the time associated with Rick's accident. Otherwise, we'd surely drift apart and get divorced. The fear of divorce gave us the motivation we needed to do something.

So, we decided to take a vacation in the Paris of North America just before Christmas because that would be really different. Luckily, my sister offered to take care of our kids that weekend.

The psychologist also advised us that it would be really beneficial for us to kickstart our sex lives into action again. His shortcut was for us to use Viagra, and he helped us get a few pills from one of the doctors using it in a study. He was quite progressive, as he also knew about the on-going studies showing that it was beneficial for women. So, he advised me to take half a pill at the same time Lewis took his to help me get into the spirit. After all, it had also been a very long time for me to have gone without any sexual activity.

Viagra, Sex, & Romance

Our first night in Montreal was beautiful, as the city was cloaked in snow and the Christmas lights were sparkling everywhere. We went to an excellent French restaurant, got a good night's sleep at our elegant hotel, and visited many charming stores and museums in the downtown area the following day. We didn't even try having sex yet. We were just having a nice time.

During that second day, Lewis began talking to me again as if I were a real person. He began reminiscing about previous trips he had made to Montreal when he was a young engineer. I enjoyed those stories about his youth, and as he talked about his topsy-turvy adventures, he began to smile. That night, before leaving our hotel, he said, "Eleanor - what do you think about taking those blue pills later tonight?" I was relieved he was even thinking about it, so of course I agreed.

After dinner in an Italian restaurant which had delicious smells of steaming olive oil, garlic, and basil, Lewis reached over and held my hand. He said, "I'm grateful that you stuck with me all this time, Eleanor. I know I wasn't the most pleasant person to be with." I think that made me feel more in love with him than I had since the previous Christmas. Over coffee, we took our Viagra.

We walked out past a department store called Ogilvy, where a crowd was pressed against a large window display of little electronic animals performing different jobs in a Christmas village. Lewis hugged me tight and kissed me in a way he hadn't done for a whole year. I told him, "I know we belong together, Lewis, and I'll always be there for you."

The smell of a wood fireplace drifted out from a cute little nearby bar, so we went in. We sat down on a sofa in front of the fireplace, snuggling together, sipping on brandy and watching the flames. Lewis kept his arm around me the whole time. Something was definitely happening within me, and I guessed within him as well. I was having both romantic and sexual feelings, and my body was yearning to be touched in a sexual way. As we got up to leave, Lewis kissed me tenderly on the lips and hugged me tight. I practically started to cry.

We had a beautiful hotel suite looking out towards the mountain, and we opened the curtains to watch the city's lights sparkling though a fairy-dust snowfall. While standing there at the window, we began deep French kissing with our tongues entwined and toying with each other inside our mouths. Lewis' mouth felt hot and eager on me, and I knew he wanted me and needed me. I felt like we were becoming lovers again. Lewis pressed up close to me, and then I felt it clearly - his erection was stiff and pointing upwards into me, as if it needed me to touch it. My heart was beating fast and I was remembering how it felt when my vagina was anticipating having his nice hard cock inside me.

Lewis and I took off all our clothes and lay down on the crisp, clean sheets with our arms around each other. He was caressing my back, my ass, and my thighs. He rubbed his face into my breasts, moaning with small sounds of pleasure. His cock was so hard, it was amazing. I knew it wouldn't go soft, no matter what. I felt it pressing against my belly and my thighs as he caressed me, and I took it in my hands and squeezed it and stroked it.

My vagina was hot and expectant, with a desire of its own to have that penis inside it. Lewis began running his fingers through my pubic hair and then rubbing my clitoris in long, soft strokes as if he cherished me. It was the first time in a year that he had done that to me, and I felt like I was a woman and a wife again. He reached a long finger inside me, and I put my hand on top of his and pressed his finger harder into me, driving me to a sexual high. But my body wasn't quite used to his touch, and I wasn't ready yet to reach orgasm. It had been far too long since he had helped me have one.

I pushed him over onto his back, and leaned towards his hard prick and put it in my mouth. His began moaning in pleasure, louder and louder, as I sucked him and stroked him. I really wanted to make him have a wonderful climax, hoping it would help to release him from all the pain and anxiety of the past. And, I wanted to start feeling like I was truly the wife and the woman he had needed for so many years. I didn't let him turn over to screw me, I just kept sucking and stroking him. He continued pushing his fingers hard into me, caressing my hot, lubricated vagina and clitoris until I was inches away from coming myself. Suddenly, with my mouth deep down to the base of his cock and my tongue tickling his tiny slit, his erection began pulsating, then shooting up hot gooey come deep down my throat. There was so much of it I gasped. I just swallowed as fast as I could. Lewis' whole body was quaking, and his hips were lifting as high as possible off the bed so that his cock could press hard into my mouth.

Lewis began crying.

I moved up beside him and I put my arms around him, and rocked him. I said, "shhh, dear, don't say anything... it's okay... everything will be okay..." I was glad he listened to me, and didn't try to talk. All the communication we needed at that point was non-verbal, and we lay together mute for 15 minutes, listening to the muffled sounds of Christmas traffic rolling by below us on Sherbrooke Street.

Lewis got up slowly and went to the bathroom to splash some water on his face. He walked back into our darkened room, and stared out the window for a couple of minutes before coming back to me in bed. I could see his silhouette, and he once again had an enormous erection sticking out in front of him. He must have been reading my mind, because he lay down beside me, and began caressing my breasts and vagina again. I had lost my feeling of sexual readiness for a few minutes, but it returned almost instantly, and this time my hips began undulating as my vagina sought to find its fill.

I instinctively raised my knees and he knelt between my legs, squeezing his erection right into my vagina. I opened up to him almost immediately. I was so excited, my vagina couldn't stop quivering around his cock. He made deep, steady thrusts into me, and he felt so much like the Lewis I used to know. At that moment, he desired me and needed me - and that was what I longed to experience.

I began digging my fingers into his back, and then I slid my hands down towards his butt, and squeezed him tight to pull him harder into me. In between thrusts, I reached between our glistening legs and caressed his testicles. My clitoris had never felt so stimulated before, and soon I couldn't stop myself from throbbing against the base of his penis as I started climaxing in fast, aching bursts of pleasure. My orgasm pulsated from deep with my soul through my vagina, releasing me from so many months of physical and spiritual frustration.

Lewis kept screwing me even after I came because he wanted to have a second orgasm. He soon was released again in climax, and then he sighed deeply and turned over to relax on the pillows. We were both exhausted by then, and we pulled the sheets over us and slept in each others' arms, totally isolated from the outside world.

At breakfast the next morning, we began talking some more, and we mentioned Ricky's name for the first time in days. But it was different. Now, we were allowing ourselves to let each other into our hearts, and to heal our wounds. The bond that was being renewed gave us strength to look forward to the future, to start treating ourselves and our other children in the most positive way possible.

Corrie was going to need braces, Jason needed encouragement to keep up his grades, and Rosanne was trying to get into med school. All three needed our support and our strength. And Lewis and I needed to begin living our lives again. We resolved that day to turn a page towards the future.

Our highlight that day was getting a lot of physical activity. We went ice skating indoors in a rink at the base of one of the downtown skyscrapers and then had a steambath and swim at the hotel's health club. That really made our stress melt away, and we were very ready for intimacy as soon as we got back to our hotel room.

That time, I don't think we even needed any Viagra, but we decided to take some anyway just to avoid the possibility of disappointment. It kicked in as we were lying around watching TV, as we both became very sexually oriented. My vagina started having that pulsating, desiring quality, and Lewis' erection was clearly pushing up against his sweat pants.

Lewis helped me take off my track suit, and he stared up and down at my naked body in the window light. I'm glad I still have a pretty good figure, even after the four kids. He had me kneel down on the floor facing the snow-dusted window, and he began screwing me from behind while we watched cars and people rushing about far below us. His cock went hard into me, and I tilted up my ass so that his tip would squeeze against my G-spot with each thrust. My vagina was very aroused, so it was really erotic to have his hard cock inside me again. He reached around my thigh and caressed my clit in his hands. This time I climaxed before he did, and it made me shudder as if I was being tossed in a tidal wave of pleasure. I reached behind me to touch Lewis and feel him close. Then, I began to fondle his balls the way he likes, and he came after a couple of minutes, ejaculating deep into me.

Lewis had a great idea. He said, "Let's not go out tonight, Eleanor, let's just lie around together and order room service..." We had a nice hot shower, then stayed totally naked as we watched TV, snuggled together, and napped. We were happy together, just lying around and doing nothing.

On our last day there, we took a ride on the subway line to try it out and to get to one of the big department stores downtown. A train was just pulling out, crammed with Christmas shoppers.

A face from inside the subway turned to me and looked at me as it sped off. The person, a teenager, was smiling, and I think through the blur of movement that he was waving to me. The weird thing is, *it was Ricky* - or at least someone who looked just like him. I gasped as I turned to Lewis: "Did you see that?" I asked.

"I think I did," Lewis replied, his voice trailing off.

We'll never know who or what that vision really was. But the important thing now is that Lewis and I have come to accept that our child always knew we loved him, and he knows our thoughts were with him every moment of his life. And, perhaps, one day we all really will be together again. I do think he'd be happy knowing that we were able to find love again, and that we're still walking down the path we chose so many years ago when our first son was born.

* * * * *

Karen's Tango Trio

CHRIS AND I WERE MARRIED ten years ago, and it was the second marriage for both of us. His first one lasted five years; mine, all of one-and-a-half years. Both of us came to realize that marriage wasn't about fairytale intentions, it was about wanting to be with someone on a daily basis.

I admit I was disappointed with my first husband because I was totally immature. I expected him to be lovey-dovey with me all the time, to bring me flowers, and treat me like a princess – as if that was all I needed to make me happy. Well, that stuff quickly wore out a few weeks after the honeymoon. Those superficial things aren't enough to hold people together.

As for my new husband, Chris, he said his previous marriage was so boring it made him want to cry. He tried to make up for the lack of intellectual stimulation on the part of his wife by having a separate life of his own. He'd go out with his baseball team pals, or with his friends from work once or twice a week, and his wife would hit the ceiling. But she had no alternative to offer him except more of her inane conversation about clothes and relatives. They ended up with one son, and they share custody. Chris and I haven't had a child because we're so wrapped up in our activities and our work, but we still have a few years left to decide. He's 45 and I'm 37.

I wanted Chris and myself to build a vibrant, on-going type of marriage that would grow and develop as we did from year to year. So, we were always open to trying out new experiences together, and we both thought that was great. It was during one of those experiences that Viagra came into play in a way that surprised both of us.

The kind of things we've been doing over the years included skiing, taking tango lessons, learning to scuba dive, and playing in a doubles tennis league. All this, along with both of us holding full-time jobs, makes for a pretty active and stimulating life. Chris would say, "Karen, this is one of the reasons why we'll always be happy with each other - because we're growing together and spreading our horizons together." I was sure he was right.

We had our strange sexual adventure while we were taking our tango lessons. Most of the people in our class were women, which seems to be the case with most dance schools. That meant there never were quite enough men to come and learn the complicated steps. Some boyfriends might visit the studio once or twice, but when they saw that they had to really think and remember what to do, they quickly dropped out. We women often danced with each other, taking turns leading. This also meant that my husband was always at a premium as a partner, and he took turns leading the women across the floor. Some of them were quite sexy. He admitted that a few of them did turn him on to some degree, but he always added that, to him, I was the most attractive one there – and I believed him. The trouble was that *I* was the one who began to get attracted to one of the women students!

I've never had lesbian tendencies. I do have several close girlfriends whom I've known for years and whom I love dearly. They've stuck with me through thick and thin from high school to college to divorce and are as close to me as sisters. I certainly never got into anything physical with them, nor did I want to. But, during our 12-week tango course, one of the other women students became very special to me. She was a lovely, chestnut-haired, brown-eyed girl named Janice with an hourglass figure and a great British accent. Her most memorable features were her pearl-white complexion and her big, innocent, smile. She wore arty-looking round glasses and seemed about 30. She told us she had dumped her boyfriend when she left England, so she obviously wasn't gay either.

Whenever I was paired up with her, we'd hold each other lightly around the waist as we did the tricky steps, such as twisting the bottom part of one of our legs around the other's leg. We'd talk and give advice to each other as we danced, and I loved hearing that cute accent of hers whenever she spoke. But more than that, I began to love the feeling of holding her in my arms. It was an entirely different sensation from being with a man. Her pastel beauty, slim waist, and shapely hips and breasts made me want to hold her in both hands like a fine porcelain figurine.

Usually, our dance group went to Starbucks after class for some coffee and dessert. Somehow, I always found myself sitting beside Janice. I didn't really care what Chris or the rest of the group would be talking about, I was always so engrossed with Janice. I found myself touching her as often as I could, and I was sure she was going out of her way to be physically close to me. Once, on our way to the restaurant after class, we trailed behind the others and actually held hands as we walked. I kept telling myself, *I have to stop thinking about Janice and picturing her face and lips in my thoughts... I'm in love with Chris, it doesn't make sense to be so taken with Janice...* But I could hardly stop myself. She had somehow wormed her way right into my heart, although I have no idea how it happened.

I decided I had to tell Chris about my attraction to Janice because I wanted him to know and maybe to help me understand it. I've always felt I could talk to him about anything, and this was no exception. He thought it was unusual, saying, "I couldn't imagine myself becoming so close to any of my male friends. But, in terms of women, if there's anyone that's really attractive, it's Janice. And, she gives off great vibes. At least you have good taste." When Chris and I made love that night after talking about Janice, it was especially hot. It was as if both of us had a need to prove how much we cared for each other.

As we approached the end of our 12 weeks of classes, our teacher announced we were all invited to her loft for the final session to party the night away. We were all supposed to dress up as tango dancers, and it seemed like we were all going to have a marvelous time. Janice and I talked on the phone at least ten times that week, discussing what we were going to wear, how we'd be doing our hair and make-up, and what we thought the men were going to wear. I think we were both happy to have a good excuse to talk to each other so often that week, and I felt really warm and close to her.

Party night rolled around, and Chris and I got really dressed up. I put on a black low-cut top with a flared black skirt, black tights, and black pumps, while he wore a black suit, black shirt, and white tie. We were quite the striking couple. Janice showed up alone wearing a dark red silk blouse and skirt outfit with red high-heeled pumps. She looked totally amazing with her alabaster skin framed by her dark red outfit, and I found my heart beating because I was so excited to see her and be with her that night.

There were a lot of arty dancer types – both male and female – at the party, and a lot of drinking was going on. We all took turns dancing with each other, and, for me, the most exciting part was dancing with Janice and holding her close to me and feeling her holding me close to her. Whenever our breasts rubbed against each other, we both seemed to prolong the contact, so that we could feel each other's nipples pressing together through our blouses. But I felt I wanted more, and I sensed she did too.

The men were drinking and talking to each other near the table with the alcohol. When Janice and I sidled over, we overheard them talking about Viagra. One of the guys said he was taking it, and pulled out his bottle. The other guys – along with Chris - acted really macho, saying they didn't need it. But this fellow said everyone should try it to find out what they were missing.

Something made me say to Chris, "Why don't you try it? Let's see what the fuss is all about."

Janice, standing beside me, also started egging Chris on, saying, "Chris – maybe you can take Karen to places where she's never been before!"

Chris looked at us both. He said, "What the hell!" and popped one into his mouth. I think he did it just to prove he wasn't chicken. He added, "I know nothing's going to happen because all my equipment works so well already."

Then, one of the guys dared me, saying, "Karen - what about you? It works on women too, you know. And all you need is half a tab." What could I do? I had already dared Chris into taking it, so I took one of the tabs and split it in two and swallowed it. On a lark, I handed the other half to Janice.

She swallowed it also.

I didn't know what, if anything, to expect. But we all acted cool and went back to the dance floor.

Chris took turns dancing with a few of the women, including me and Janice. She quickly came over to me after their dance, and said, giggling, "Dahling, I simply must tell you that Chris has an enormous erection – I could feel it several times against my thigh!" She and I laughed a bit about that, and when I danced with him next, I saw it was obviously true. I told him, "Don't worry, dear, I'll take care of that for you later – but please don't scare any of the other women with it!" and we both laughed. We figured we'd leave soon.

The music wound down, and Chris said he wanted to "take a leak", so I accompanied him down the hall to find the guest bathroom. The main bathroom was being occupied by someone smoking a joint or something, and we found the guest bathroom adjoining the spare bedroom at the end of the hall. Chris added jokingly, "Don't tell anyone, but it'll take me longer to pee than normal because of this erection!" Someone was already in the john, and, when the door unlocked, out popped Janice. I said, "I guess it's your turn, Chris - we'll wait for you out here."

Janice and I slumped down on the bed to wait for him to finish. As she lay beside me, I could feel my heart pounding. The two of us began caressing each other's arms and hair. There was tremendous electricity between us. I don't know why, but I was aching to kiss her on the mouth, hug her, and feel her in my arms. I felt utterly horny and sensuous in every part of me. Janice must have felt something too, because she was caressing my legs with light strokes of her fingertips as we lay there. I have no idea why we did this, but our faces got closer and closer, and suddenly my mouth was right on hers. Our lips were pressing together, and soon I felt her warm breath as our lips slightly parted. Our tongues met timidly for a fleeting moment, and I cherished the wetness of her saliva when it touched the tip of my tongue. I wanted to taste her tongue deeply within my mouth.

We heard the toilet flushing, and Chris came out. Janice and I both acted as if nothing had happened, although we both knew a monumental line had been crossed. I found myself telling him, "Come sit down Chris and relax a moment. I'm beat from all that tangoing and it's so nice and quiet in here." He sat down beside me and sighed deeply, and I leaned over and kissed him on the mouth and he eagerly kissed me back.

Chris didn't seem to mind that Janice was there, and, in fact, it seemed to me that her being there was turning him on. It certainly was turning *me* on. I was craving more from Janice, and she must have been reading my mind. She began to touch my back and caress my legs, and I thought I was going to go crazy. I lay above Chris, kissing him as Janice stroked my legs and my butt behind me, in a way that Chris couldn't see. She then flagrantly reached her hand right under my skirt, pulled down my tights, and began caressing my bare ass and thighs. The touch of her hand on my naked skin made my hips start to squirm - and that really got Chris going. I could feel his cock pushing up at me from inside his trousers.

I undid his zipper to pull out his boner, and he grasped my hand for a moment to stop me - but then he let me continue. I exposed his beautiful erection, which looked equally as beautiful as every other erection of his I've ever seen, Viagra or no Viagra. However, this hard-on did turn out to be longer-lasting. His penis was very hot, and I began to suck on it while Janice leaned against my back, rubbing her breasts on me, and playing with my ass. She soon slid her hand down between my cheeks to my pussy, and rubbed my vagina with her fingertips. Then, when she saw how crazy I was becoming from her touch, she inserted a finger into me. It felt as if my whole body was blushing from my sexual yearnings.

While still sucking on Chris's hard-on, I reached one hand behind me into Janice's red silk blouse, and slid my fingers down into her bra and onto her soft breasts. I began stroking them and caressing her nipples and enjoying every minute of it. I had never touched another woman's breasts before, and it felt more beautiful than I could have imagined. As I was kissing Chris's steel-hard erection, I could feel Janice change positions so that she was leaning over to face Chris - and she begin kissing him on the mouth. He seemed to be enjoying it - me on his cock and Janice on his mouth - and I wasn't jealous at all. This was such a fantastic new sexual experience, I just wanted to go along with the flow – at least for this one time.

Janice slid her hand down, and she began playing with the shaft of Chris's cock while I sucked the crown of it. I could feel her fingers slipping into my mouth along with his penis from time to time, so I licked them as well, and ran my tongue over her long nails and fingertips. I had never been so turned on in my life! Chris started stretching his hand down to stroke my pussy, and he was surprised to find my panties already down to my knees. He rubbed my clitoris and pushed one of his fingers deep into me. A moment later, Janice's hand was also rubbing my pussy, and she inserted a finger into me right beside his, and then they both had their fingers and hands all over my vagina. They were rubbing the outside of my pussy, my clit, my G-spot, my vulva, all of me. I could barely stand it anymore, and, a moment later, I began climaxing in convulsions. There was no stopping me – or my two sexual partners.

I took off everything I had on the bottom, and so did Janice, and the two of us pulled off Chris's pants. He quickly pulled off both of our blouses and bras and stared intently at all of the breasts that were within his reach now. He fondled Janice's and my breasts at the same time, seeming to get a great deal of enjoyment. I wanted Chris' magnificent erection inside me, so I straddled him and began fucking him deeply as he lay on his back. His cock was firm and hot inside me, and I moved my hips up and down as I fucked him in a rocking motion.

Janice kneeled beside me, and she and I put our arms around each other. Finally, I was able to feel her mouth on mine again as she began French-kissing me. She pushed her sensuous tongue forcefully into my mouth, and it was a delicious feeling to have her with me face-to-face like that. With her tongue in my mouth and Chris' cock in my vagina, it was quite the peak experience.

Janice reached down to the junction of Chris' cock and my cunt, and she began toying with both of us at the same time. She rubbed his cock and my clitoris with each stroke of her hand, making my pussy feel as hot as steam. She squeezed and tickled my vulva in a way that only a woman can. Meanwhile, her ass and pussy were totally exposed and practically rubbing against Chris's face. From her kneeling position, she lifted her leg up and over Chris so that she was straddling his chest while facing me. She and I continued kissing each other as she leaned her hips backward towards Chris, then lowered her ass and pussy down to his mouth. He began licking her pussy from that strange upside-down angle, and I made a mental note to try it myself one of these days.

It was Janice's and Chris's turn to climax, and they both did at almost the same moment. Chris's erection inside me began vibrating and quivering, and he shot out come like a volcano. He was groaning and practically screaming with his mouth against Janice's pussy in a way I had never heard him do before. That was exactly when she came herself. I felt it happening as her lips parted and she sighed in hot, long breaths against my face. She didn't stop rubbing my clit with her fingers and palm, pressing even harder as she came, and I found myself climaxing again, in beating pulses of excitement.

We all flopped down on the bed and lay there in a heap of nakedness and sweat, all of us trying to get our breath back. I was in the middle, and I put one arm around Chris and the other around Janice. None of us was embarrassed, although I guess we should have been.

Chris opined, "I blame it all on the Viagra."

Janice and I quickly agreed, even though we all knew it was just a good excuse. A few months have passed since then, and Chris and I are still really happy with each other. In fact, we're planning to have a baby. We've never had another one of those adventures. I doubt that our night of crazy passion could ever happen again. Janice and I talk to each other from time to time, but our lives haven't reconnected since the tango lessons ended. She's planning to return to her boyfriend in England. I appreciate having such a great husband - and the fact that he was able to let us both play out our adventure without having any admonishments.

The End

Viagra, Sex, & Romance